Dr. Angela Fetzner

The wonders of woodland

Translated by
Phil Stanway

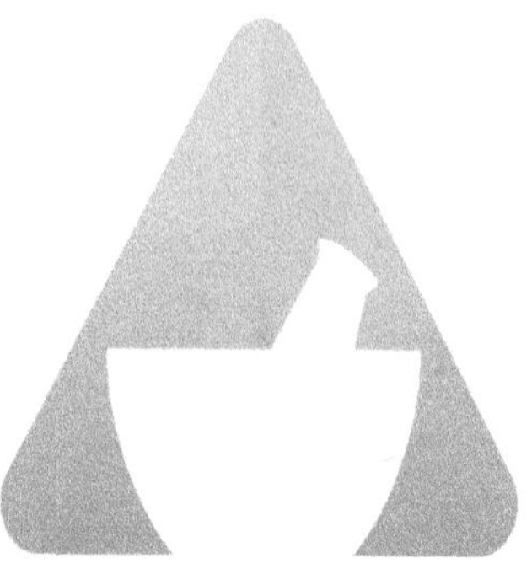

Imprint

Translation by Phil Stanway
original german title „Im Bann des Waldes"

Coverdesign:
ZERO agency, Munich
using motives from shutterstock.com
Coverphoto: © kdshutterman depositphotos.com
Book set: Michael Raab

ISBN: 9798655313507
Imprint: **Independently published**

Contents

„The clearest way into the Universe is through a forest wilderness "

(John Muir)

Woodland – a contemplative site

Exposed to a flood of sensory impressions and an ever faster pace, more and more of us are finding it hard to switch off and relax, but at the same time, there is an ever growing need to slow down and recover.

The more we yield to the burden of multitasking and succumb to the stress of hobbies and rushing around, the more we need an alternative and counterweight to the challenge of modern times.

As life becomes more hectic and demanding, we often long only to let go, empty our minds and let ourselves drift.

Too many appointments, rivalry at work and strife in the family – far too often we are caught in the tread-mill of must and should.

In woodland, we are free to roam and dream without any obligations and to observe without interfering. We can impartially let it affect us and note the effects.

There is no competition or pressure to stand out in woodland; there is no agitation or deadline to be met.

We leave the vicious circle of doubt and reflection, and instead we feel and live in the present, in the here and now.

We escape the vortex of negative thoughts and worries, and the primal force of woodland takes over, offering us sustenance, strength and consolation.

Our hearts dilate, our minds become free, and we change from thinking to feeling. We breathe the power of the woodland in without impairing the woodland in any way.

Nature draws us away from our worries, vexations and problems, and our minds focus on nature and trees, becoming more attentive and meditative.

With increasing technology and digitization of the world, we long for the simple and unadulterated, the calmness and seclusion of nature. We long for what is intelligible, for a safe haven in troubled times.

Woodland offers this and much more; it is first and foremost a place of power and the epitome of continuity and stability. It offers a refuge from sickening events and serves as a shelter for the restless and troubled soul.

In woodland we are left with basics and experience the essence and genuineness of life.

We learn again that true happiness comes from within and can be experienced only in the here and now.

We learn again to appreciate the blessings of the moment and to value simple things, offering new insights.

In woodland we especially feel part of nature and symbiotically connected. The boundaries between nature and humanity blur, and the transitions are no longer noticeable. We feel safe, at peace and serene, suffused with a deep contentment often lost in everyday life.

We no longer have to think, reflect or plan; we are simply alive, have arrived and are connected with woodland, as by an invisible but lasting bond.

Anger and grief, shallowness and trifling fade away, shamed by nature's beauty and power of healing, and lapse indefinitely into the background.

Woodland offers the soul a home and a haven, where it can freely recover.

Woodland grounds us, as the deep-rooted, lasting trees strengthen us, empower us and heal us on all planes.

The trees' roots lead us back to our own, letting us feel firmly in place and secure in our lives.

We have a chance to rediscover our true selves.

But of course, such awareness is possible only if we open ourselves to woodland and yield to the powers of nature, since only then do we have moments of deep tranquility and delight and inspiration.

Woodland offers a path to our real, original and pure selves. Otherwise, far from nature, merely sitting around and consuming what is offered, we gradually lose touch with our real potential. Television, Facebook and Instagram draw us away.

Often, we lose ourselves in superficiality, vanity and banality, neglecting deeper values.

We have to realize that we ourselves are the obstacles in our paths, not this or that in the world around us. We prevent ourselves from evolving and finding the path to our true selves.

We have withdrawn from nature's riches and beauty not only around us but also within us. We merely wish to fit neatly into society and to keep up with the latest trends. We even tire ourselves out through leisure activities, as if keen to hide from our own gaze.

Many of us would like to know ourselves better but find only an inner emptiness, so we try to be busy at all times, to avoid the inner emptiness and sadness. We would rather face a flood of new events on television or find a new way to kill time with other people.

We are unable to keep company with ourselves and to be alone. We need other people to amuse us in breaks or to leave us no time for dark thoughts, as we have few close friends whose company we really value.

Even in company, we are not really present, we do not really heed the people facing us or listen to their problems or worries. Instead, we heed the beeps from our portable phones, letting us know that messages through WhatsApp are urging waiting for answers.

In trying to be accessible on all planes and to dance at all weddings, we end up being nowhere and having no real affections.

And if we happen to be anywhere, our thoughts have already moved on to another place.

It is easy enough to realize that under these conditions we rarely feel really happy and that any happiness felt is fleeting.

Woodland grounds us again; it lets us feel the real purity and beauty of nature.

In woodland, we begin to relax without thinking about it, and our jittery nerves calm down. Everyday life with its schedules and locations becomes unreal, and the goodwill of nature goes to our hearts. We feel peaceful, easygoing and in harmony with everything around us.

By taking a little time off from civilization, we gain fresh vitality and energy. In the stillness of nature we regain our inner balance.

We are alone but no longer lonely; we are not sad but at peace with the world.

Being alone in a wood does not transform us into shy hermits, bitter outsiders or misanthropes. Even the most sociable person needs to be alone at times, to regain enough vitality to cope with civilization.

Being close to nature, we refill our reserves of energy, feel less stubborn and resentful and regain our sense of humanity.

In woodland, we again become aware of ourselves as wholes, not merely as a potpourri of roles and habits – thorough and precise at work and more flexible and casual at home. Woodland reassures us and invites us to open our eyes.

In woodland, we are brought back to the here and now; we appreciate the world around us and are grateful for what it is and for what we are. Woodland enriches us in all respects; we experience it anew every time, and this feeling of novelty then embraces the whole of nature and ourselves.

Nature is our anchor. It encourages us to be kinder and more attentive to ourselves and others and to the world around us.

Woodland receives us as guests. It does not grade us, comment on us or make demands. It has no expectations but takes us just as we are, each of us a unique human being.

Woodland grows and helps us to grow too and to become more positive, whereby we become more stable and rooted. In this respects too, woodland is exemplary.

Woods as the earth's lungs

Like greenery in general, woods have an ecological function and can be understood as being the lungs and metabolism of the earth, which has created not only leaves and flowers but also animals such as humans. We humans are a part of the earth as an organism. Owing to its special qualities, humankind has created so-called civilizations and has set itself apart from nature. Like a cancerous growth, it acts not only in its own interest but also against the interests of many other parts of its own organism. It fells trees and woods, deals with other creatures as it happens to feel fit and exploits the whole earth for its brief gain.

For awhile, this may seem to work. As the so-called crown of creation, humanity proliferates like a tumor at the cost of the earth's health and that of all earthly creatures, by spreading into and ruining whatever parts of the organism are still intact. But the sad reality is, that with the death of the whole organism, the proud tumor of humanity dies too.

The natural world of plants is more cooperative. Plants breathe on behalf of the earth and all life, offer shelter and nourishment and create a natural balance. Every single plant makes a contribution, but the overall effect is due to their cooperation, as in a huge swathe of intact woodland.

Little primeval woodland is still around us. It has been forced to make way for cultivated trees and plants, but in spite of human intervention and often poor behavior, woodland is still enchanting. As long as parts of it are still intact, the ruinous behavior of humankind will not ruin the innate vitality of plants and woods.

This vitality is no longer evident to all people. They have closed their ears and eyes and are no longer able to sense the throbbing of life in every tree.

Trees linking heaven and earth

Trees are rooted in earth, but their trunks reach for the sky, and their branches, twigs and leaves are keen to embrace the sun. if it rains, some of the drops are caught by the leaves, but others fall or trickle to the earth. Substances dissolve in it then are taken in by roots and passed on to the trees as a whole. Some moisture then evaporates from the leaves and rises into the air to form clouds, completing the cycle of events. Twigs, leaves and fruit fall to the earth, where they decay and enrich it with their nutriments, so trees are always part of a natural cycle.

In drawing nourishment in through their roots and using it for growing towards the sky and the sun, trees also create a visible link between heaven and earth and are part of their interaction.

In mythology, the connection between above and below, between heaven and earth goes further. The world-tree is a symbol of life and also of the cosmos, encompassing the world above, the world below and the material world in between. This is also a link between life on earth and the other side, which appears in various religions as heaven or hell or as the realm of the gods of the upper and lower worlds.

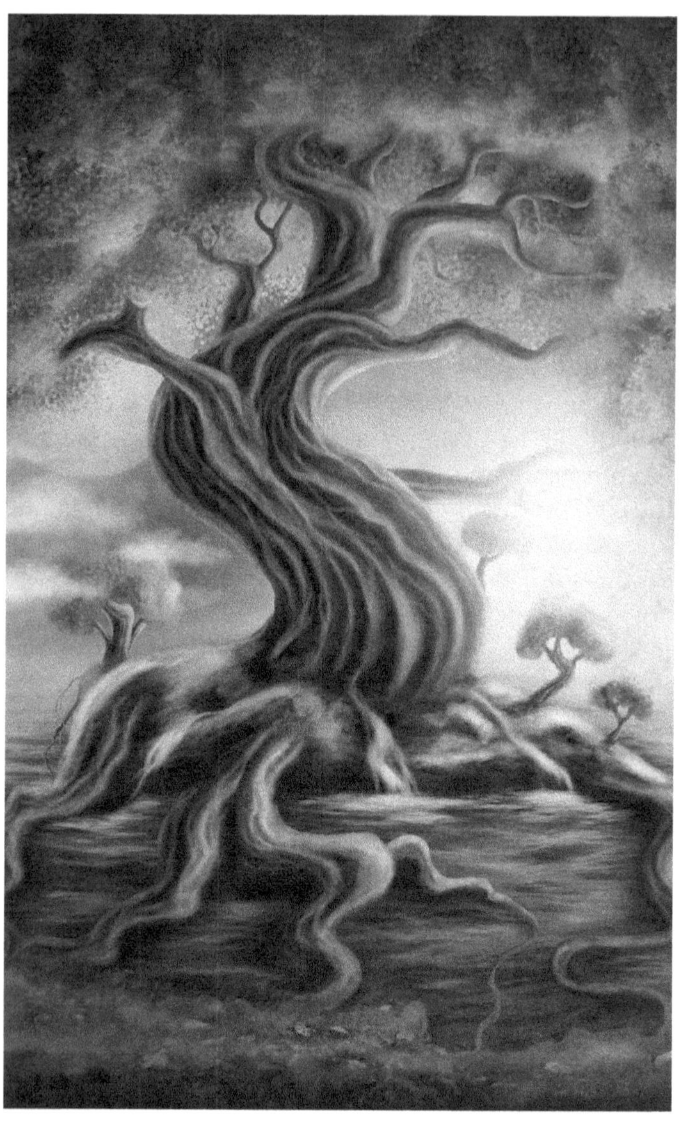

© depositphotos - egal --- The world tree belongs to the mythology of many people and is an ancient symbol of the cosmic order. It is at the center of the world axis. It connects the three levels of heaven and earth and underworld.

In linking worlds or in standing for existence as a whole, the world-tree also stands for all creatures, including ourselves, in the upper and lower worlds and thereby for the whole of life.

If you walk into a wood, you may fail to realize that there is much more life around you than your eyes are able to see or ears to hear.

There are plants and countless organisms and woodland spirits. The trees and plants are full of inner vitality. Like all other kinds of life, they are able to interact and communicate with their surroundings, but every tree is also self-sufficient like all other plants throughout nature. All plants have the specific qualities and powers they need. Moreover, the flora as a whole forms a network, including not only all plants but also all other life in the woodland.

Hardly have we entered a wood and immersed ourselves in its restful ambiance, lush greenery and fresh air than our moods change. Worries and vexation fall from us as lightly as drops of dew, while stress and responsibilities gently dissolve. Everyday life becomes unreal and loses its urgency and soon fades into the background.

We become part of a symphony of hues, sounds and scents interwoven into a harmonious and peaceful composition as appealing to our hearts as to our minds.

The woodland replaces worries, sorrows and sadness with an eagerness to absorb its soothing variety. We pause, amazed and grateful, relishing the present moment for all it is worth.

The focusing of our attention on the essential, on the here and now and our own being, grants us authentic and intense experience and may lead us to view things differently and to find our real nature, which is all too often lost in the treadmill of life.

The attention we pay to woodland is neither deliberate nor forced upon us; it is effortlessly achieved without any ulterior motive. Here we notice a stone decked in moss, and there we see the ground carpeted with wood anemones.

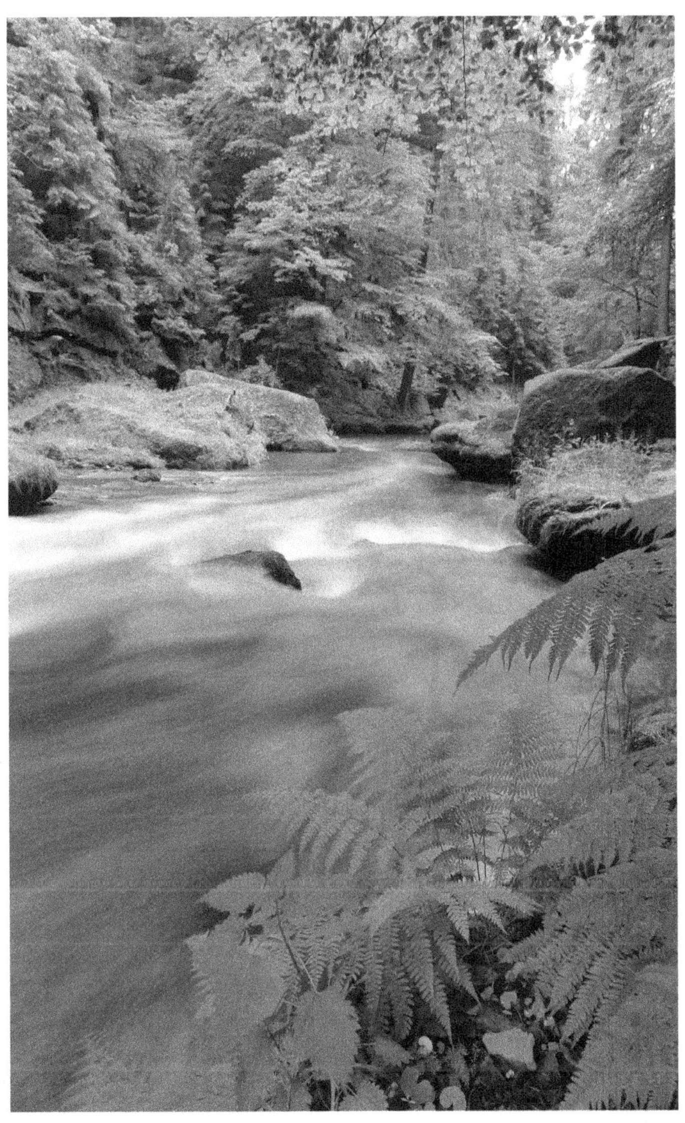

© depositphotos - rdonar

Woodland

The pale sun of spring shines up at us out of a pool. On breathing deeply in, we scent the moist earth, the decaying leaves and the fresh moss, intermittently revealed by the interplay of light and shade.

We pause to view the trunk, branches and cones of a spruce, scenting the essential oil and the tree's height and firmness. At one with nature, we relax wholeheartedly, sharing the deep peace and harmony. Strolling along with a meditative state of mind, we achieve rest and inner balance. Thoughts melt away, as we view the beauty and preciosity of nature, which enchants us again and again.

Moments spent in woodland in the midst of nature are unique. There are always new impressions, which nature never wearies of conjuring up.

We appreciate every tree, animal, plant, flower and even beetle, as we tread carefully, to avoid harming any.

In woodland, we feel like home-comers, not visitors. We feel sheltered and on intimate terms with our surroundings and able to be as playful as children.

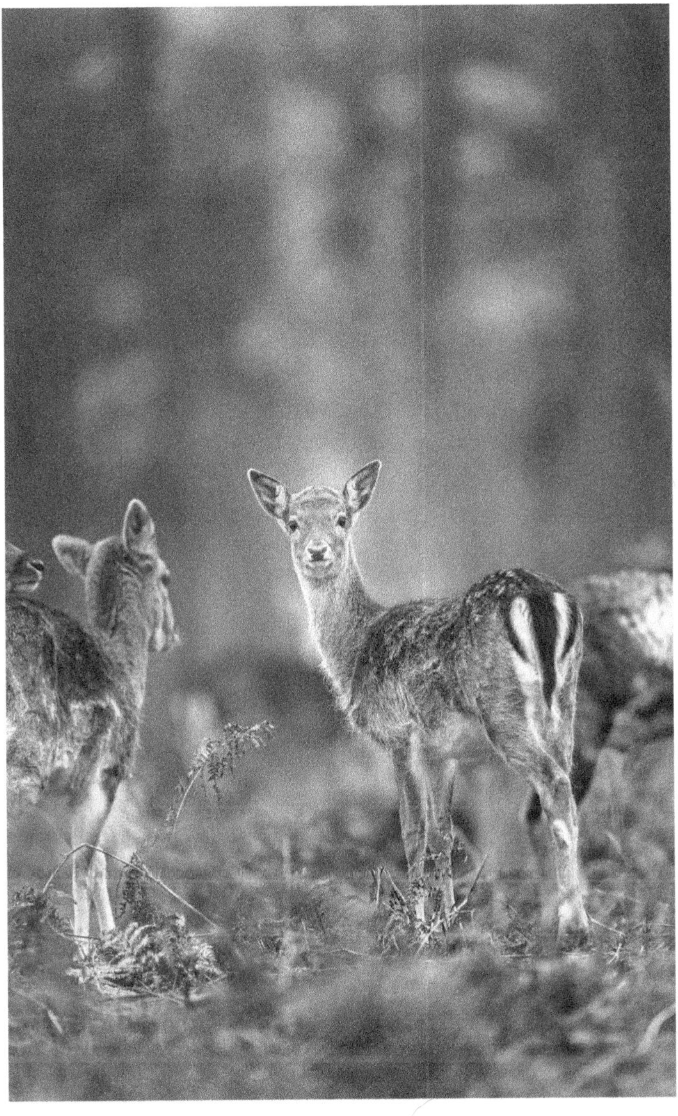

© depositphotos - ysbrand

Deers at woodland

The scents in a wood reawaken long dormant memories of childhood and carefree existence, as scents leave deeper impressions than other sensations.

The wind ruffles our hair and the coolness reddens our cheeks, as a few raindrops fall from the trees and moisten our faces. Soon the sun reemerges and warms our skin and our hearts. We breath in a mixture of scents from coniferous branches, resin, moss and leaves.

Under our soles, there is no hard asphalt but only the light and springy loam. We are drawn further into the woods, where sounds fade, damped by the trees. We stroll into the undergrowth and walk over stones and toppled trunks.

Everywhere there are gentle sounds, of twigs crackling underfoot or the soughing of foliage. They are mostly discrete and soothing. The woodland vibrates, being full of life and motion. Ants scurry hither and thither as busy as builders.

There is movement everywhere but also rest. We immerse ourselves in a sea of hues and sounds, as if floating in a bath under only the open sky.

Sometimes rain suddenly gushes down with a rumble of faraway thunder. The wind whirls freely around us, smelling of spices, ruffling the ferns but not the moss and roots. This is something for us to enjoy, as it sweeps old cobwebs away. It is so much bigger than we are and treats us as parts of a whole. No longer do we feel empty and isolated but involved in a living world.

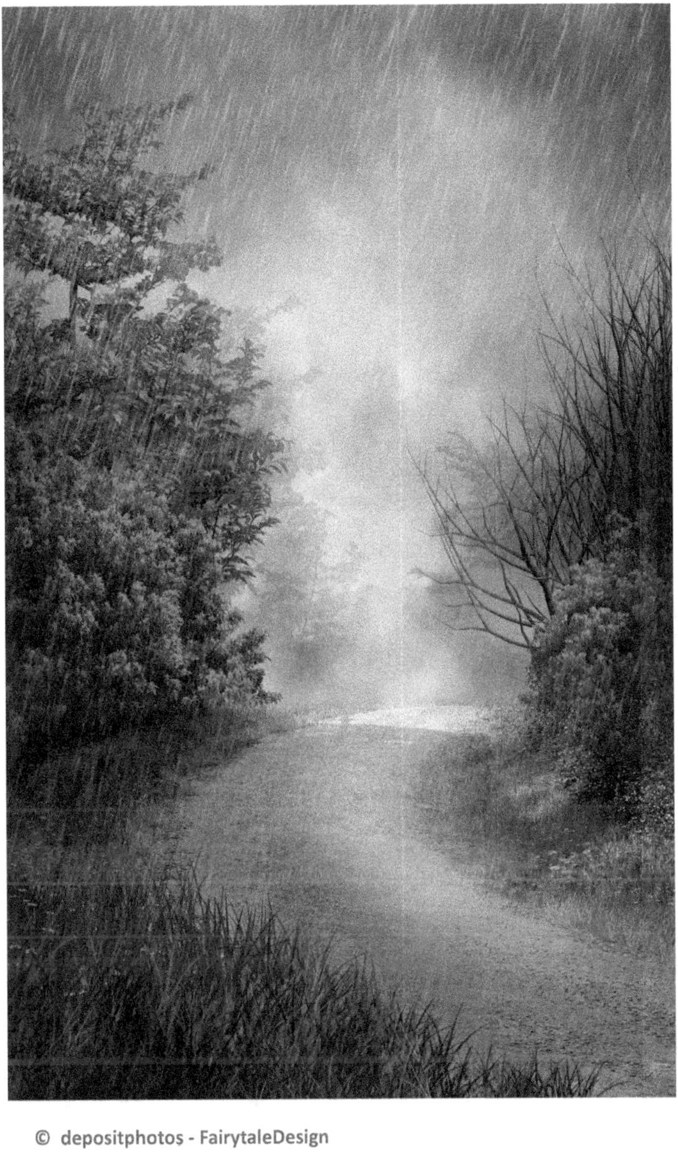

© depositphotos - FairytaleDesign

Rain at woodland

The trees beckon us to pause and admire their rich variety of shapes and hues.

The light is gentle, the stillness palpable, and the burbling of a brook reveals its presence. We loosen up and are invigorated by the fresh and cool air.

Birds twitter, leaves rustle, beasts scurry and trees sway. We pad over soft moss, as sunbeams brighten a clearing. The scent of wild garlic and the musty smell of mushrooms rise from the earth and mingle with the scent of elder-blossom.

How lovely it is to see brown spruce needles and dry leaves on the ground. Nature is so varied, inimitable and beautiful! Our senses are neither overwhelmed by new impressions nor deprived of any. There are fresh sounds and scents and all the hues of the rainbow, and nothing is quite as expected. It is neither too much nor too little.

Nature furthers our feeling of well-being and soothes our nerves. The trees, the plants and animals are a unique selection and miracle of creation.

Peace is all around us and within us, while civilization is kept safely out of sight. We are alone but not lonely. Our resilience and powers are renewed, enabling us to cope with everyday life on our return.

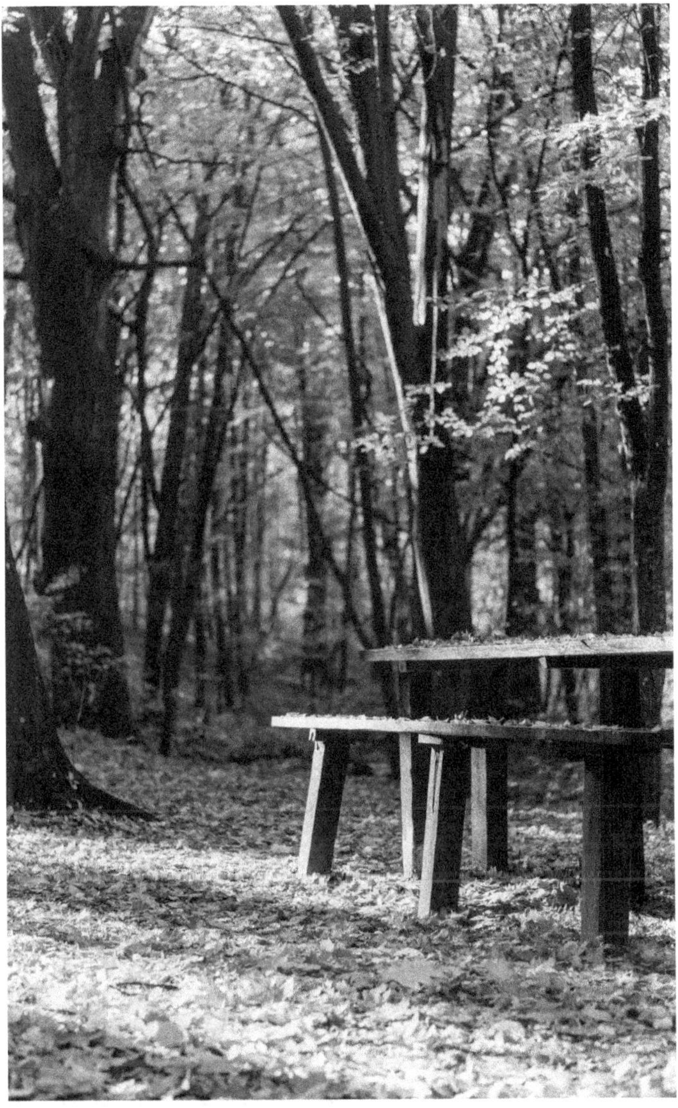

Woodland - a place of rest and reflection

It is not selfish of us to withdraw from the madding crowd at times; it is only a sign of accepting responsibility for ourselves and our peace of mind. We have to pay some attention to ourselves and to leave the superficiality of everyday life behind.

We are simply drawn by the tapestries of woodland and the songs of hidden birds and would like our lives and theirs to be intertwined.

Relaxation occurs naturally in woodland, as the place is pleasant and picturesque, encouraging us to slow down and take it easy.

We become less tense and restive and more aware of ourselves and our needs.

The greenery calms and soothes our spirits as much as our eyes.

Natural sounds like the songs of birds and the burbling of brooks tell us: More haste, less speed! Life should be enjoyed, not finished by 5 o'clock!

The seasons of our lives may adapt to the seasons of woodland.

Spring is like childhood and youth, summer like full maturity, fall like the ripeness of age, and winter like resting in peace.

But one cycle of the seasons leads to the next, and winter to spring and so on. There is continual change and transformation but also continuity and consistency.

Our lives are as transient as nature as a whole, but the spring of hope continually returns with the promise of life and renewal, a world without end.

Dalliance in woodland also shows that happiness does not have to be sought afar but is often lying in wait, a few lanes away. We have no need to trek to rumored regions, bearing our tents and supplies, or to hire special equipment for nights in tropical jungles. Nature is more than willing to meet us half way, if we only let it.

We have no need to book package tours to the other end of the earth. Nature is here and now, within walking distance. We just have to heave ourselves up onto our feet and stroll off.

Woodland is deeply at peace with itself and a more suitable part of nature than most for sharing its peace with us in our spare time.

Woodland is alive with all kinds of creatures, continually interacting and relying on each others' achievements.

Trees warn each other of the nearing of bad weather or harmful insects, and birds warn each other of the nearing of predatory birds.

Fungi live symbiotically with trees, and some fungi and algae live symbiotically as lichen, so woodland may be restful but it also a place of continual interaction and interdependence.

We too may interact by cautiously getting to know it better, expressing our appreciation and fellow-feeling.

Body and soul come to rest, resentments fade into the background, and cares become inconsequential. Nothing remains to vie with the honesty, integrity and authenticity of nature.

The wonders of woodland

In fantasy films, trees sometimes appear as characters like the *Ents* in The Lord of the Rings.

The film *Avatar* showed very nicely how all plants in a wood are related and communicate with each other. Indeed, such a network of plants and trees has now been scientifically investigated. The fact that this has hardly been mentioned in the media may be due to the realization that it has little practical or commercial value. But in other respects, this interdependence has a lot to teach us.

As living beings, plants are more deserving than most of us willingly admit. On seeing stems, branches, trunks, blossoms and fruit, we merely realize that plants need water, light and nourishment.

We may also know that they change carbon dioxide into oxygen through photosynthesis. Plants and trees are a prerequisite for the survival of all other creatures, for without them, there would be no usable air or greens to eat.

But is this really all there is to them? Druids, shamans and nature-healers are convinced that even the tiniest plant has a life of its own, consisting of much more than mere growth and chemical processes, providing animals such as ourselves with the needed foodstuffs.

Nature-lovers are also aware of trees' enchantment and view each wood as an organism, whose organs are flora and fauna. We need only stroll into woodland and be open to its powers and inhabitants, seen or unseen, for them to accept and help us.

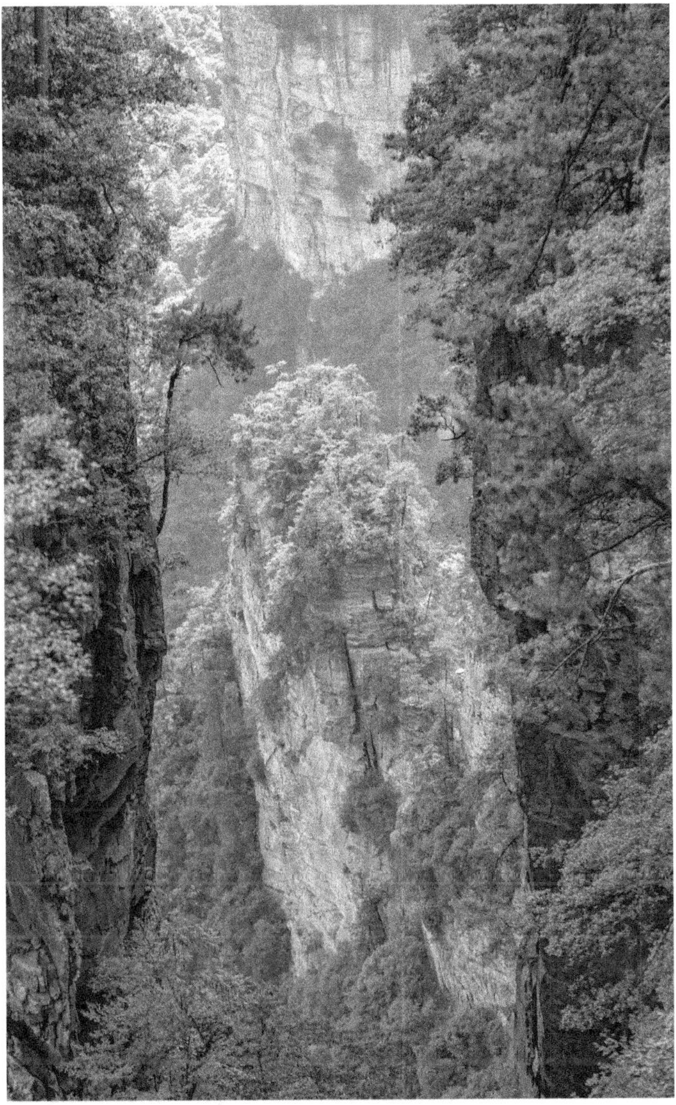

© depositphotos - pawopa3336

Pillars of heaven with trees and woodland similar to the landscapes in the movie „Avatar"

27

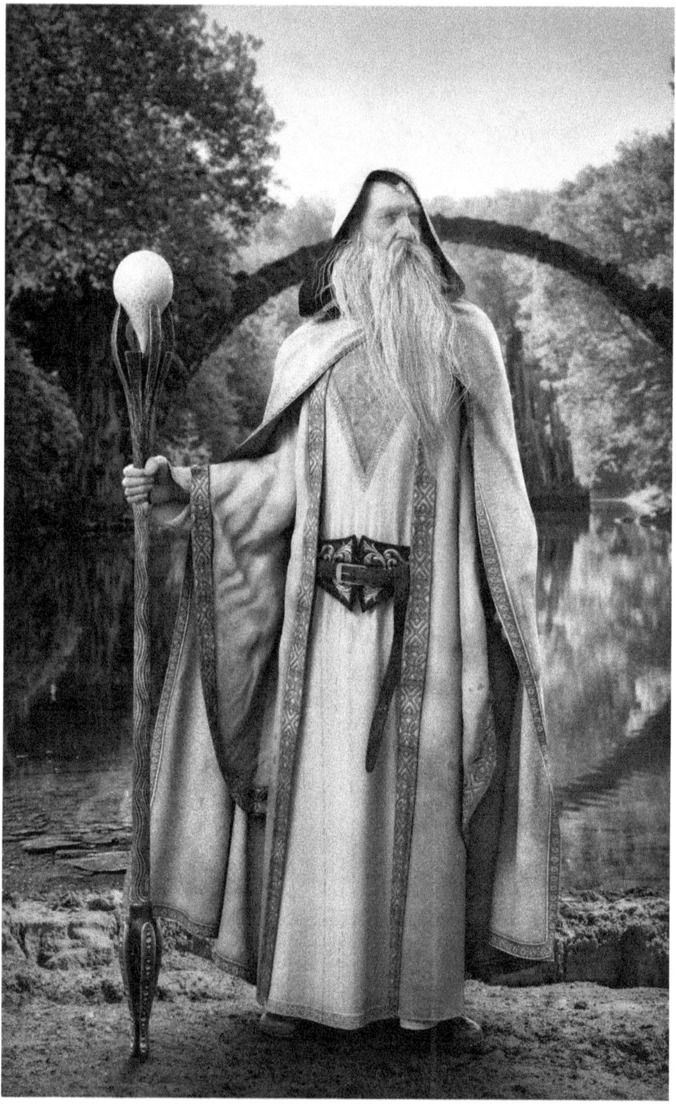

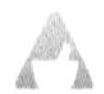

© depositphotos - digitalstorm

Druid at woodland

The language of trees

Trees are holy. Whoever is able to speak with them and to listen to them has access to truth. They preach no sermons or platitudes but, without pandering to any individual, they preach the original principle of life. **(Hermann Hesse, 1877-1962, writer and painter).**

Trees have no ears, no vocal cords, no mouths and no eyes, but they continually absorb and react to information from their surroundings. Their sense organs are their roots and leaves, as initiates close to nature have always believed, and as scientists have recently confirmed. Trees communicate with each other and interact socially.

The research has been carried out by scientists at universities in various countries. They have found that trees are continually taking information in through their roots, assessing and reacting to it. Even Darwin referred to roots as trees' brains.

The tips of roots make their way through the soil like worms in seeking water, moisture or nourishment or avoiding poisons and so on, as these are all relevant to trees. The information received is passed on through the trunks to the branches, twigs and leaves, who react in terms of growth.

This explains why trees shut their pores in periods of drought. They thereby protect their resources of energy and live longer in limiting the loss of water through their leaves by evaporation.

At the same time, the shoots and leaves take information in about their surroundings and pass it on to the roots.

If infested by pests for instance, the shoots and leaves tend to spread an alarm. According to the kind of pests, a tree produces more substances to repel or kill them.

Oak leaves and acacia leaves produce more tannin, as this is toxic to some of the pests eating them.

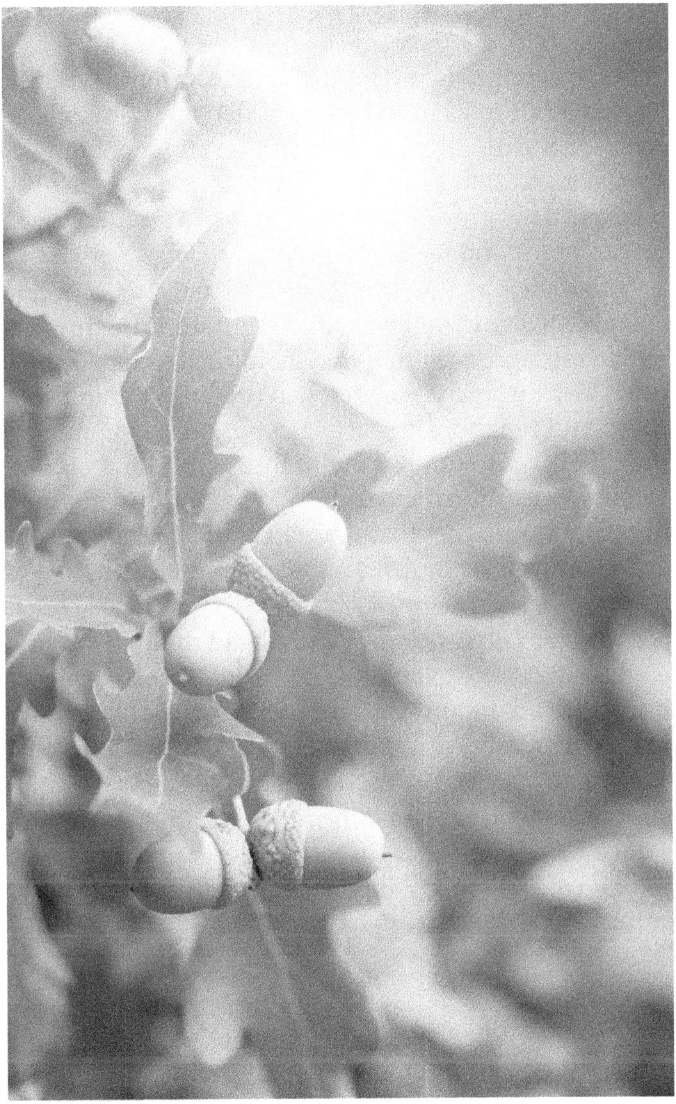

Oak leaves and acorns

The communication of trees

A tree has not only its own system of defense but also alarms other trees in the event of danger. For instance acacias produce more tannin and release more ethylene. On sensing this ephemeral substance, trees nearby increase their production of tannin, as a South African researcher found out.

A researcher at the University of British Columbia was able to show that trees also communicate through their roots and even that they help each other reciprocally. For instance, if a tree has too little mineral nutrient and neighboring trees have more than enough, they let it have some of theirs through symbiosis between roots and fungal networks. The networks free important nutrients from the soil, then are offered sugar produced by nutrient absorption and photosynthesis.

The fungal network may pervade a whole wood and enable all plants to interact. This interaction consists not only of communication but also of vital measures like deliberately supplying needy trees with nutrition. Trees and plants have also developed effective and subtle strategies. Research into wild tobacco for instance has shown that the plant reacts to being infested by caterpillars by increasing its production of nicotine.

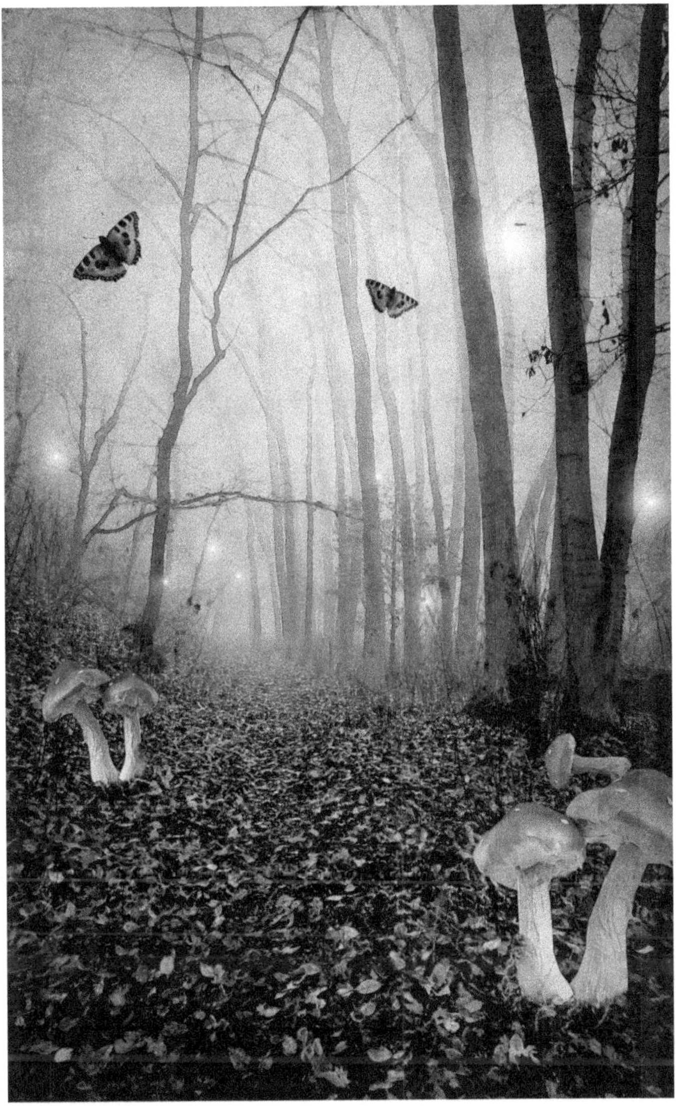

© depositphotos - hofhauser

Symbiosis trees mushrooms and other plants

If these defensive measures prove to be inadequate, the plants release certain scents, to attract creatures who feed on caterpillars, but this is done only if there are too many caterpillars, for a certain number of butterflies are later needed for pollination.

For this reason the caterpillars are firstly drawn to the plant by a scent. Only if the caterpillars endanger the plant, by eating too many leaves, does the wild tobacco try to hold them back by releasing more nicotine or by attracting ants to act on its behalf. These are only a few examples from science and research, to show that trees have means of communication and mutual help, of self-defense and self-preservation, which they are able to use strategically. They resort to specific measures to solve specific problems, and they identify problems by processing sensory input.

But trees' ability to communicate goes much further, as they are also able to communicate with us.

Communicating with trees

Trees are unable to use words, so a normal conversation with them would seem to be impossible. If we wish to understand them, we have to open our senses, heed our thoughts and feelings and our bodily reactions.

Many of us know well enough that dalliance in a homely garden with plants appreciated and looked after has a relaxing and freeing effect. Likewise, in strolling through woodland, we are freed from everyday stress, and the restfulness of the woodland spreads through the whole of our bodies.

Just walk into woodland, to experience it for yourself. Find out what effects the various trees in the area have on you personally and record your experiences. You have no need to be a druid or shaman, to become familiar with the language of the trees.

In fact, there is even no need to sense something consciously, to be enriched by the trees, as this happens more or less automatically. Just as trees act on their own behalf and on behalf of their fellow trees, the trees have a positive effect on your feeling of well-being, your health and your powers of recovery. This is due partly to the beneficent ambiance of woodland working on your body and mind, making you more resilient and stress-resistant.

At the University of Vienna for instance, it has been found that our pulse slows down and our blood pressure falls or becomes stable in woodland. Even muscles may become more relaxed.

One of the things which you measurably receive in woodland are so-called phytocides. These are substances which trees produce and release for the sake of protecting themselves. They have an antibiotic effect and encourage our bodies to synthesize killer cells, to fight pathogens there. This greatly supports the immune system, so between trees in tended woodland and us, there is a genuine give and take as a kind of communication.

Conscious communication

Just as biological and chemical processes can be stimulated in woodland, as shown by phytocides, there are exchanges in other areas.

Sensitive measuring instruments show that trees react in various ways to harmonious or threatening surroundings. If for instance, we approach a tree with ill intent, the tree is able to sense this as clearly as a neutral or openhearted friendly approach.

A tree with its web of roots in the earth and its trunk and crown in the air can be thought of as a complex radio station with receivers and transmitters. Trees are continually receiving signals from their surroundings and sending signals out, so their thoughts and feelings can be measured as waves.

We likewise receive signals from our surroundings. Just as eyes receive beams of light or ears receive waves of sound and put them together as images or chords, we receive signals which may neither be seen nor heard but sensed and experienced.

Let your eyes wander through the woodland. Is there a tree, which you especially like and which somehow appeals to you? Do you feel drawn to one tree more than to another? How do you generally feel among all the trees?

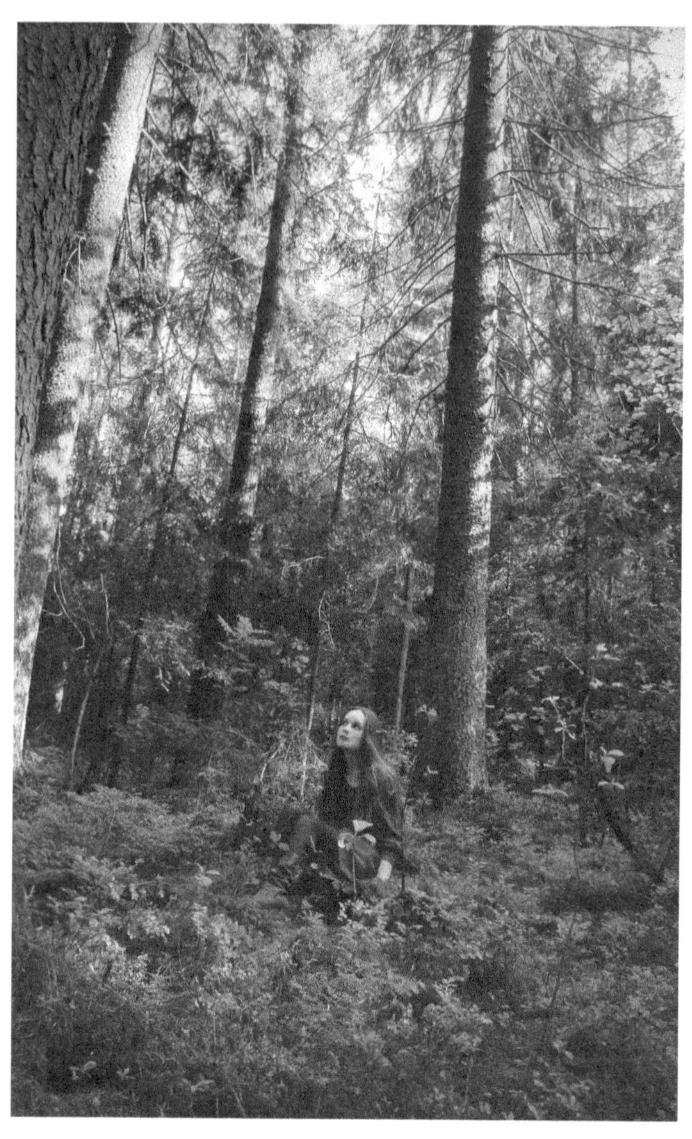

© depositphotos - aliftin

at the bottom of woodland

Choose an attractive place and settle among the trees, then as they work upon you, heed the impressions.

You can also choose particular trees and get in touch with them in the following way. You begin by greeting a tree chosen and run your hands over its bark, then if you feel welcome, you embrace it. Feel its energy, the flow of life from its roots in the earth up to the uppermost twig and back.

Heed what goes on in yourself. Maybe you feel protected, energized, joyful or something else. This is a communicative exchange of energy. The tree makes its nature known to you and senses your own nature. It may even offer you a gift like a falling leaf, twig or fruit.

You may bring some water with you and grant the tree a little. Often what are welcome are positive feelings, for instance in the case of a sick tree.

Feeling like a tree

Instead of trying to get in touch with a tree directly, we may resort to exercises and kinds of meditation, to familiarize ourselves with a tree's qualities. One of these exercises comes from yoga and is called 'the tree'.

The yoga exercise 'the tree'

What place could be more suitable for practicing *'the tree'* (vrksasana) than woodland? A tree is rooted deeply in earth, and even if a gale blows, the tree is more likely to sway than break. Likewise, the yoga exercise *'the tree'* bestows more resilience and confidence on us and leaves us more restful and energized.

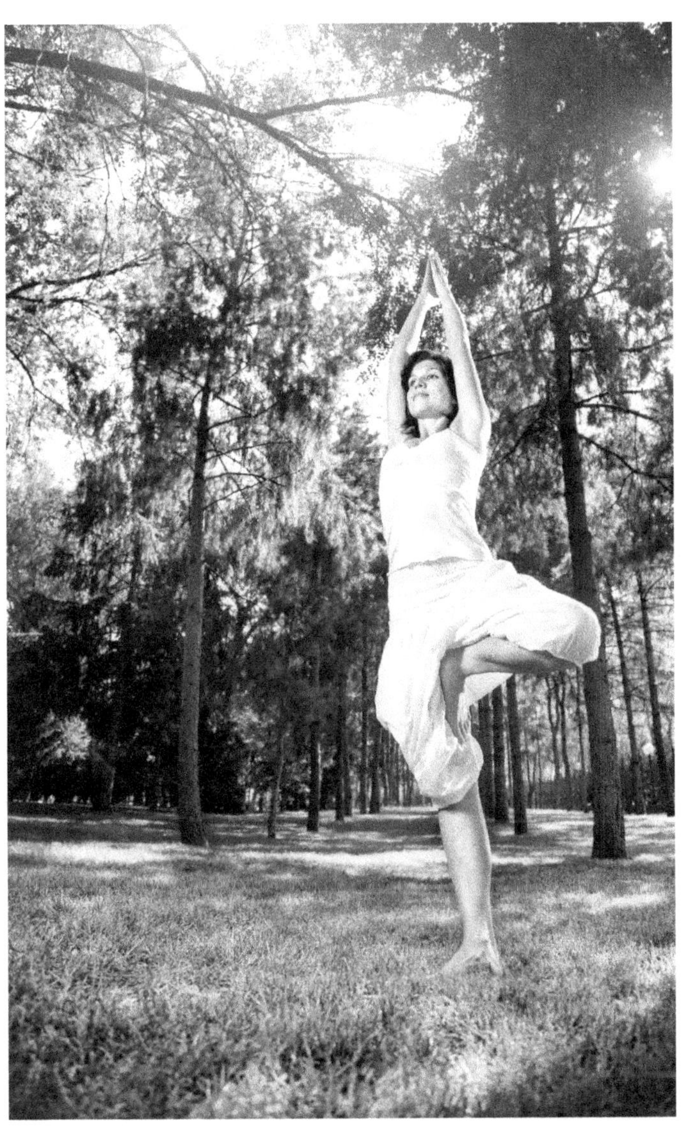

© depositphotos - byheaven
yoga exercise
‚the tree'

- Stand straight up and keep your feet together. Take several deep breaths in and out. On breathing in, feel how the energy of the earth flows into you, and on breathing out, feel how it flows out of you again.
- Bend your left leg to one side and place the sole of its foot against your right leg for support then draw it up till it rests on your right thigh. At first you may feel rather wobbly, but remember you are like a tree and that energy is flowing through your right leg.
- Lift your arms, slightly bent, above your head till the palms of your hands come together over your head. The upper part of your body is like the upper part of a tree, taking in energy from the sky. In yoga, this pose helps us to feel more rooted, at ease and in touch with above and below. Stand firmly on the ground but loosely, not stiffly.
- Hold the pose for about 15 seconds.
- Repeat the exercise with the other leg.
- The exercise **'the tree'** strengthens our sense of balance and improves our posture. Mentally, it helps us to be more purposeful and decisive.
- Practice this exercise regularly and feel what it is like to be a tree.

Alternatively, you can imagine what is happening inside a tree in front of you, how it experiences standing in one place and how energy and force flow through it. Try to feel its ambiance and vitality. Lean back against the tree while sitting or standing there and feel its life. You may like to ask it to share with you some of its restfulness and energy. Finally thank it and get used to treating it respectfully.

If you feel rebuffed on nearing a tree, respect that too, as all creatures like to be left in peace at times.

If, on the other hand, you feel accepted, you may be able to make friends with the tree. Heed your heart and let your positive feelings or your love and appreciation flow to the tree. Also be open towards the tree, to receive whatever the tree would like to communicate in return.

Some people receive images or symbols and others receive certain emotions, moods or spontaneous thoughts. The important thing is to remain unprejudiced and as open as an inquisitive child.

Practice this with various trees and you will find that the communication or exchange feels different in each case.

The contents vary according to a tree's personality, as they do in the case of smaller plants too, as they differ as species and individuals.

Further exercises in woodland

Here we can look at a few exercises which can be practiced without much ado. They are gentle and playful but should nonetheless be practiced with an awareness of body, spirit and soul. There should also be attention to breathing, though the breath should flow freely, whether we are still or moving.

For these exercises, choose a place in the woods, where you feel at ease. Stand there casually, letting your arms hang loosely. Stretch your arms up and breath in deeply. Imagine that with each breath you are breathing the energy of the woodland in. Finally breathe out slowly and lower your arms, imagining that you are releasing the used-up energy into the woodland.

Simple circular arm movements

Let your arms move in circles, sometimes forwards and sometimes backwards then in opposite directions. Stretch your arms up then back.
Breathe deeply and attentively.

Proper breathing

Breathe in for 4 seconds then breathe out for 7 seconds. Try to practice this exercise for several minutes as training in deep breathing.

Simple practice in breathing

Shut your eyes and breathe deeply through your nose, letting your belly swell. As you breathe out, let it sink back. Observe how your breathing changes and repeat the exercise five times.

Letting thoughts drift

Shut your eyes and concentrate on only your breathing.
Breathe in deeply, savoring the power and restfulness of the woodland. On finally breathing out, free yourself from unpleasant thoughts, cares and anxieties. Let any such thoughts pass like clouds in the sky.

Breathing exercise

Breathe in and out deeply. While breathing out, squat down, till you have no air left in your lungs. While breathing in, stand up straight again.
Repeat the exercise at least thrice.

Directed breathing

Breathe slowly into your palms, as if to moisten them. Now breathe in through the nose. Repeat this exercise, till your hands have become warm.
This exercise leads to a deep and restful rhythm of breathing.

Press your lips lightly together.

Breathe against the increasing resistance but not to the point of blowing the air out. Keep your lips together and let the air pass passively out against the resistance of your lips. This will give you are feeling of how your lungs gradually empty.

At the end, breathe calmly in through the nose.

Breath out once more against the resistance of your lips. Repeat this exercise many times, till you are able to breathe freely and evenly.

The lip brake is especially useful in the case of breathlessness. It can also be used in the case of physical exertion or for relaxation.

Diaphragm breathing

Stand straight. Your feet are close together and your arms hang loosely down.

Now imagine that your belly is a pair of bellows, which puff the air out through your pipe. Now breathe in slowly through the nose and let your bellows fill with air and your belly bulge.

Breathe out calmly and slowly through your nose. Your bellows puff the air out of your lungs, and your belly becomes flatter and flatter.

Lay your hands on your belly and feel the rise and fall of your breath. Repeat this procedure for several minutes, till you feel a deep relaxation. You body is now replenished with oxygen.

Stand on the ground with your feet as far apart as your hips and your knees slightly bent and shut your eyes.

Let your weight press down equally on both feet and feel the firmness of your posture and the ground.

Imagine that you are linked to the earth like a tree. Feel how deeply your roots go down into the earth and how firmly you are anchored there.

Be aware of the stability and firmness of your posture. Breathe calmly and deeply.

Stand up straight and shift your weight onto your left leg. Breathe calmly and concentrate fully on the exercise. Now do the same in the other direction by shifting your weight onto your right leg.

Breathe deeply, keep your head vertical and look straight ahead.

If you are so inclined, you can hug a tree. Choose a tree which appeals to you, approach it carefully and get in touch with it. Hug it gently and feel its powerful energy. Breathe consciously into your feet and imagine that roots are growing out of you too into the ground. Hugging a tree brings peace, a sense of shelter, protection and comfort and frees us from restlessness, nervousness and anxiety.

Take into yourself the energy and vitality of a tree and at the same time let it bear your burden of worries. The tree will give you energy without even feeling the loss and will merely send your worries on into infinity.

Thank 'your' tree and wish it all the best!

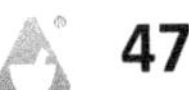 **47**

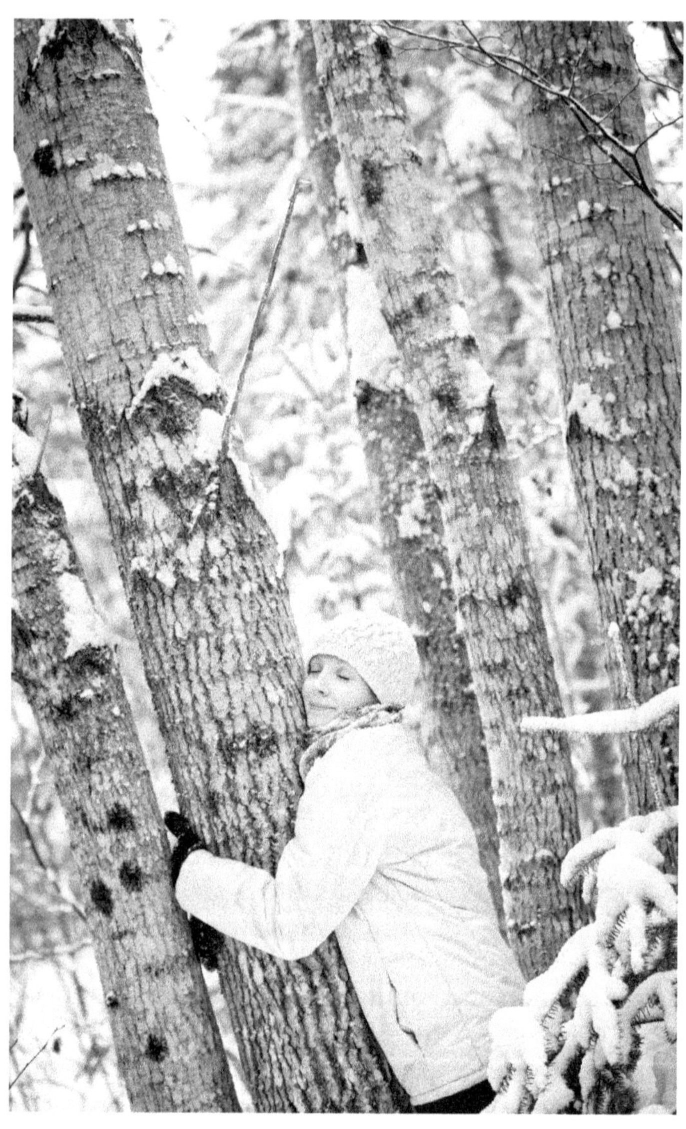

© depositphotos - aetb

Hugging a tree

Taking root like a tree

Just imagine that you are sending your roots down into the earth like a tree. You are standing firmly anchored in the earth, and nothing can throw you off balance. Be aware of your firm stance and your connection with the earth. Imagine that like a tree you are taking foodstuffs and water through your roots into your body. Feel how these supply you with energy, vitality and well-being. Stretch your arms up slowly and attentively and feel the warmth of the sun on your twigs and leaves. Notice how peaceful and relaxed you become in the course of this exercise. Breathe deeply and calmly.

Breathing consciously

Deep and regular breathing is one of the most powerful sources of our health. Deep breathing bestows vitality, equanimity and harmony and is the basis of good mental and physical health. In modern civilization, most of us have lost the knack of breathing naturally. We then have problems in moving and with the circulatory and respiratory systems as well as psychological problems.

Thus it is all the more important to learn to breathe slowly and rhythmically without interference. It is no coincidence that an important feature of breath therapy is letting the breath come and go. Breath should again be felt and experienced. Proper breathing wonderfully replenishes vitality, while harmonizing and balancing the body, soul and spirit. An interlude in woodland can help us to regain a natural feeling of how to breathe and help us to practice breathing.

If we breathe deeply into our bellies, we are more focused at work and have more vitality, perseverance and resilience.

If we deliberately breathe in deeply, the belly bulges, then as we breathe out, the diaphragm relaxes and the belly sinks back, pressing the depleted air out. A positive effect is the activation of self-healing powers, and the body is better supplied with oxygen. We feel livelier and more at ease with ourselves, and our bodies become deeply relaxed.

Calmly and evenly breathing with the belly can also improve the performance of the lungs and remove a greater amount of harmful substances.

Natural breathing is restful and relaxed and lets a person be suffused with energy. Regular breathing massages and stimulates all inner organs, improves the digestion, the metabolism and the immune system. Proper breathing is light, slow, warm and relaxed, and this is reflected by the way the body feels. Natural breathing lets us feel mentally and physically fit.

Anyone willing to heed breathing can learn how to breathe deeply and harmoniously, then energy will flow through the whole body, letting stress, tension and disharmony be reduced.

The positive effects of deep and relaxed breathing are due to its calming the vegetative nervous system.

Moreover, the proper way to breath relaxes the body, furthers equanimity and inner peace and lessens or removes many mental and physical ailments.

We can learn to breathe calmly and evenly by breathing through the nose into the belly and by breathing out only about half as fast. Both breathing in and breathing out, especially the latter, lead to deep relaxation. We should take care not to hold the breath after breathing in but to breathe out at once. Only after the whole cycle of breathing in and out should we briefly pause.

Especially in times of great stress or emotional crisis, conscious breathing is a wonderful way to find our own centers of gravity and balance and to further our inner and outer growth.

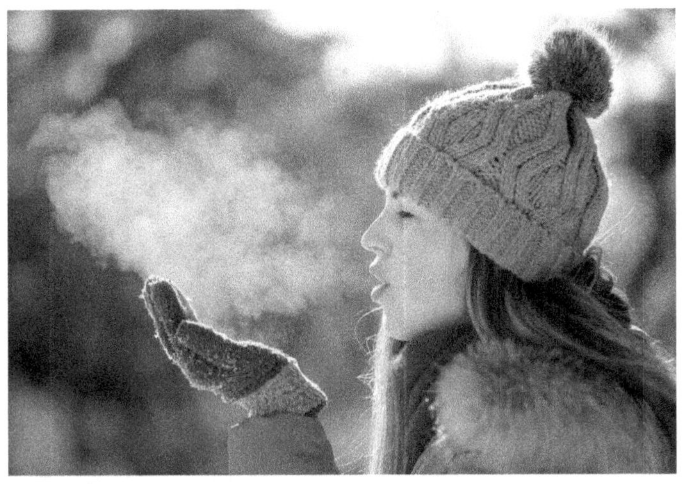

© shutterstock - illustrissima

breathe

The special effect of woodland?

Maybe you are now wondering what is special about the effect of woodland. After all, are there not other beautiful and healthy places, especially in Germany, where there is not only a central mountainous region but also the Baltic Sea, heaths, moors, lake districts, vineyards and orchards?

Every landscape and variety of nature may have its own charm and special advantages, but woodland is exceptional in having many positive effects on the health.

Woodland has many special qualities and features which support each other in the system as a whole, adding greatly to their healthy effects.

Indeed, from time immemorial, woodland has captivated whoever has ventured into it. It offers shelter and safety and a chance to shed mental and emotional burdens.

Woodland offers visitors many varied impressions, which stimulate the mind without placing undue demands on it. For instance, it offers visitors not only many kinds of trees but also a greater range of plants and animals than any other landscape or biotope. Moss, ferns, lichens and fungus all typically contribute.

Wild garlic and forest goatee are typical woodland plants, like those bearing tasty blackberries, wild strawberries and blueberries, though care should be taken to avoid eating poisonous plants like lily of the valley, deadly cherry and foxglove.

Even plants such as ivy, snowdrop, cowslip, wood vine, wood anemone, forest hawkweed, true lover's knot and burdock are integral parts of woodland, and the animals are more diverse and numerous than those of other ecosystems. Fallow and wild boar, squirrels, foxes, rabbits and mice are common features, as are many birds and insects.

Woodland has a range and variety unequaled by any other ecosystem. It is a network of plants and animals who all interact in one way or another and are thereby interdependent. Fungi for instance live symbiotically with trees, and the one partner is unable to flourish without the other. Lichens, on the other hand, are a symbiosis of fungi and algae.

Trees also send chemical signals out to other trees of the same kind and even to other trees, to warn them of imminent danger.

These chemical signals may mark their domain or inform other trees of predators or unfavorable weather. The trees thereby informed release further chemicals to keep intruders at bay.

Even birds call to others, to warn them of the nearing of predatory birds.

Thus, a wood is a place of rest but also of incessant communication.

In a wood, there is a dynamic equilibrium, a natural cycle in continual motion. Dead organic materials such as leaves are changed by fungi back into inorganic materials, which are then taken in by fungi and plants as foodstuffs.

The dead materials thereby become part of new life in a cycle of decay and regeneration.

Of great benefit to the health are essential oils, released for instance by conifers. The scent spread by spruce, fir, pine and larch is typical and wholesome. The essential oil consists mainly of terpenes, especially limonene, camphene and pinene.

For this reason, coniferous and mixed woodland are especially good for the health.

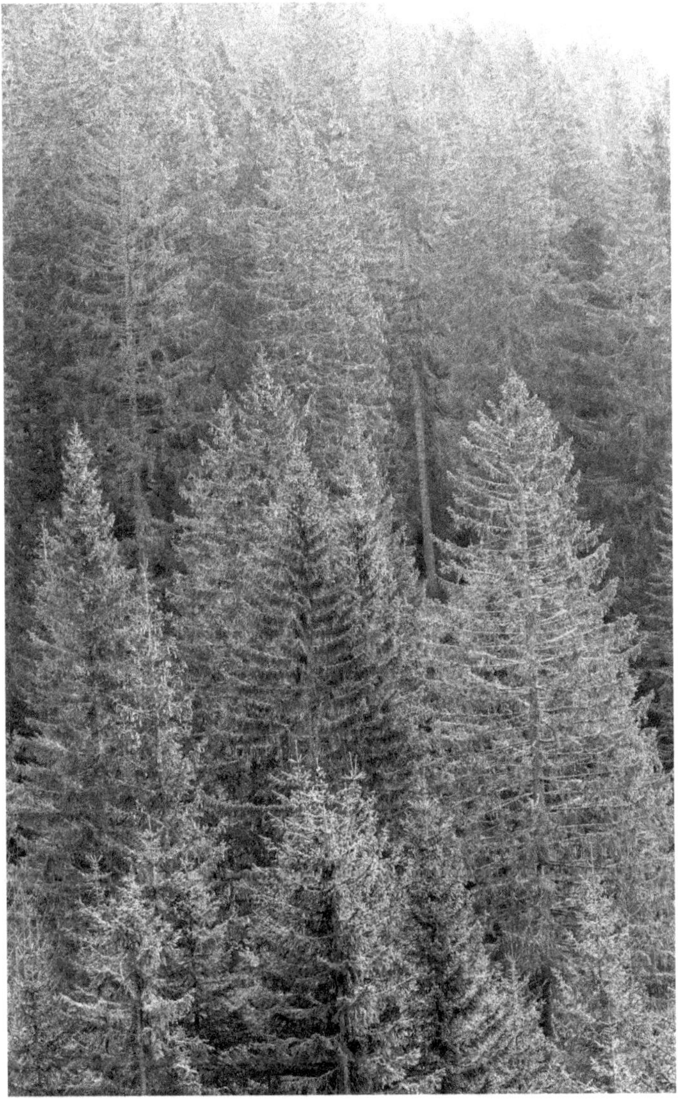

© depositphotos - zlikovec

Coniferous forest - spruce - fir - pine

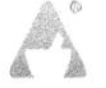 55

It has long been known that the essential oils of conifers have a healthy effect on ailments of the respiratory organs and that limonene, camphene and pinene dissolve slime, are antiseptic, antibacterial, antiviral and good against cramps.

Owing to these properties, strolls through woodland are especially good for people with difficulties in breathing, be they acute or chronic. Dalliance in woodland is good for people with chronic bronchitis, asthma or tuberculosis or inflammation of the nasal cavities.

Conifers' terpenes also help us if we are exhausted, short of energy and drained; they lessen tension, restless, stress and nervousness and bestow stability and comfort.

More recent scientific studies show that terpenes can do even more. One day spent in woodland is enough for them to increase the number of killer cells in the blood by 40% and to increase their activity by 50%. Killer cells increase the body's immunity and belong to the nonspecific part of the immune system.

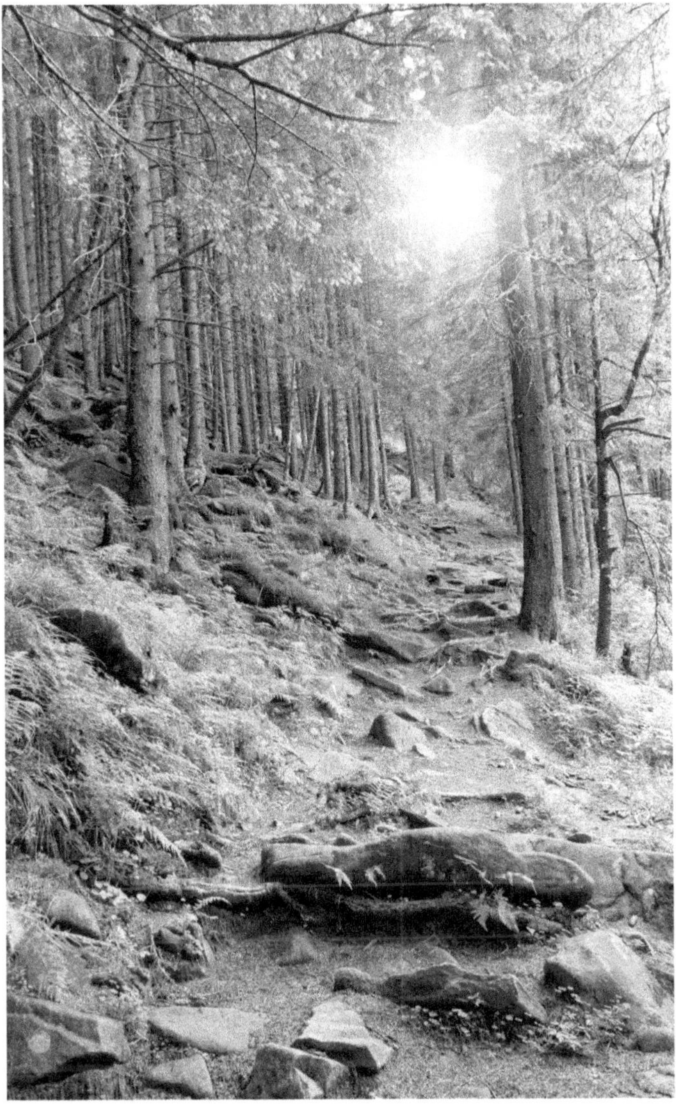

© depositphotos - pklimenko

a way in the mountain woodland

Further dalliance in woodland increases the number of killer cells even more and this increase in number and activity is measurable up to 30 days later.

There is also a measurable increase in the production of anti-cancer proteins, which help killer cells in their fight against cancerous cells.

The longer we dally in woodland, the more effective and long-lasting the effects.

The highest concentration of terpenes and other medicinal substances is in the midst of woodland, where trees stand more closely together and the air is less swiftly replaced by air from elsewhere. After rain or mist or in summer, the concentration is especially high.

Further positive mental and physical effects of terpenes and other medicinal substances in woodland are mentioned later.

A further advantage of lingering in woodland is the abundance of oxygen and the lack of pollutants. The greater number of trees and plants within the same area increases the amount of oxygen, as all plants produce oxygen in the course of photosynthesis, and they also absorb the carbon dioxide we have breathed out and render it harmless.

Dust, particles of rust and harmless gases are filtered by the woodland, leaving mainly pure air, which has 90% less dust than urban air, while harmful gases like nitric oxide are absorbed by trees. All in all, the air in woodland is like the air among mountains or by the sea in being healthier and less polluted.

Moreover the leaves and needles of the trees release water through evaporation, so the air becomes moister than out in the open. The greater humidity is a blessing for people whose respiratory organs are vulnerable or ill. A high humidity keeps the mucous membranes moister, thereby helping them to counter colds and influenza.

The higher humidity also lets the terpenes circulating freely in the air be taken in more easily through the lungs. The effect is like that of breathing more deeply. The humidity and the terpenes together have a synergistic effect.

Moreover, woodland also shelters us from the rain, cold and wind or in summer from the heat of the sun. This makes woodland a pleasant environment, however unpleasant or extreme the weather.

In summer as in winter, we can benefit from the moderating effect of woodland on temperatures. In summer we appreciate the airy and cool oases, and in winter the shelter from piercing winds.

It is not unusual for temperatures in woodland to be about 3° to 6° milder than in open landscape and to be about 4° to 8° milder than in city centers.

In place of the grey of tarmac and concrete, there is the green of foliage lavishly at hand.

Healthy greenery calms the mind down and rests the eyes. It is a hue typical of vital nature and offers hope for the future. It promises health, inner equilibrium, relaxation and harmony, and helps to lessen nervousness, irritability, sleep disturbances, anxiety, depression and sadness.

Moreover, greenery refreshes weary eyes and improves sight.

But our feet are not neglected, as the springy soil in woods is a blessing for our soles, especially if we walk barefoot. Unlike asphalt or paving stones and bathroom tiles, the ground in a wood is a surface to which our feet have naturally adapted.

Asphalt and other unnaturally hard surfaces are painful and bad for our feet, but the loam in a wood is good for not only our feet but also our bodies as a whole. Strolling on it is not a strain but massages our soles, whose reflex zones activate other parts of the body. Walking barefoot is natural, so by walking barefoot regularly, we can regain a natural and healthy way of life with consciously performed rolling movements of the feet.

Even the muscles of the feet and the Achilles tendons are strengthened and trained by continually walking barefoot. All in all, the statics of the whole body are improved by the natural way of walking, so pains in the hips or back may dwindle or even vanish.

The senses of balance and touch are likewise positively influenced, and if for instance stones tickle our feet or we feel the needles of firs, our whole sensory system is stimulated.

Walking barefoot brings us closer to nature in every way.

Knowledge of woodland

Nearly a third of land all round the world is made up of woodland, and Germany is no exception. Bavaria is the part of Germany with most woodland, but Hessen and Rheinland-Pfalz are more wooded, as woods make up 42.3% of their area.

In Germany there are 51 different kinds of trees in the woods, but 26% of the trees are spruce, 22.9% pines, 15.8% beeches and 10.6% oaks. Silver birches, common ash, black alder and European larch are likewise common.

Converting woodland and changing trees

German woodland was originally made up mostly of deciduous trees, especially the *red beech* (Latin: Fagus sylvatica). The present mixture of trees with a big share of conifers reflects the use to which woods have been put in recent centuries.

Especially from the Middle Ages to the 19th century, many woods in Germany were overused and left bare. To ensure a supply of wood, the devastated woods and bare sections were replanted along the lines of planned forestry.

The trees used for replanting were mainly the *common spruce* (Latin: Picea abies) and the *Scots pine* (Latin: Pinus abies), both of which are robust and able to cope with the difficult ecological conditions of bare areas better than for instance the red beech and silver fir. Moreover spruce and pines grow fast and yield more timber. Spruce prefers relatively moist soils, whereas forest pines manage quite well in dry soils with little nutrition.

Nevertheless, the conversion of woodland into mono-cultures, consisting only of spruce or pine for instance, has natural drawbacks. For instance they are vulnerable to the bark beetle and other insects, the soil becomes more acidic, and the risk of forest fires and wind throws is greater.

For these reasons, there is a trend towards creating mixed woodland with a diverse and stable range of trees, to replace purely coniferous woods.

Facts about trees

Common spruce

The *common spruce* (Latin: Picea abies) is the most common woodland tree in Germany, where it makes up about 26% of woodland. Its being so widespread is due less to nature than to planned forestry, as explained above. Woods made up only of spruce are seldom natural except in much cooler climes, as in Siberia or Scandinavia. In warmer climates they are more exposed to various pests like the bark beetle.

The *common spruce* may live for as long as 600 years. This evergreen tree reaches a height of 40 m and under certain conditions even of 60m.

The *common spruce* grows fast and, in being an important source of timber, is also known as the bread-tree.

In the field of medicine, oil from spruce needles is used as an essential oil and as a component of various liniments and salves.

In Germany the *common spruce* was the tree of the year in 2017.

It is used as a symbol of hope, of force, of life and vitality. In earlier times, the spruce was taken to be a feminine, protective tree, able to heal human ills by taking them upon itself.

The spruce was also used as a Christmas tree, to take the spirit of the woods into people's homes to be revered. Recently, it has become less fashionable for this purpose, as it loses its needles fast in comparison with a Norwegian fir.

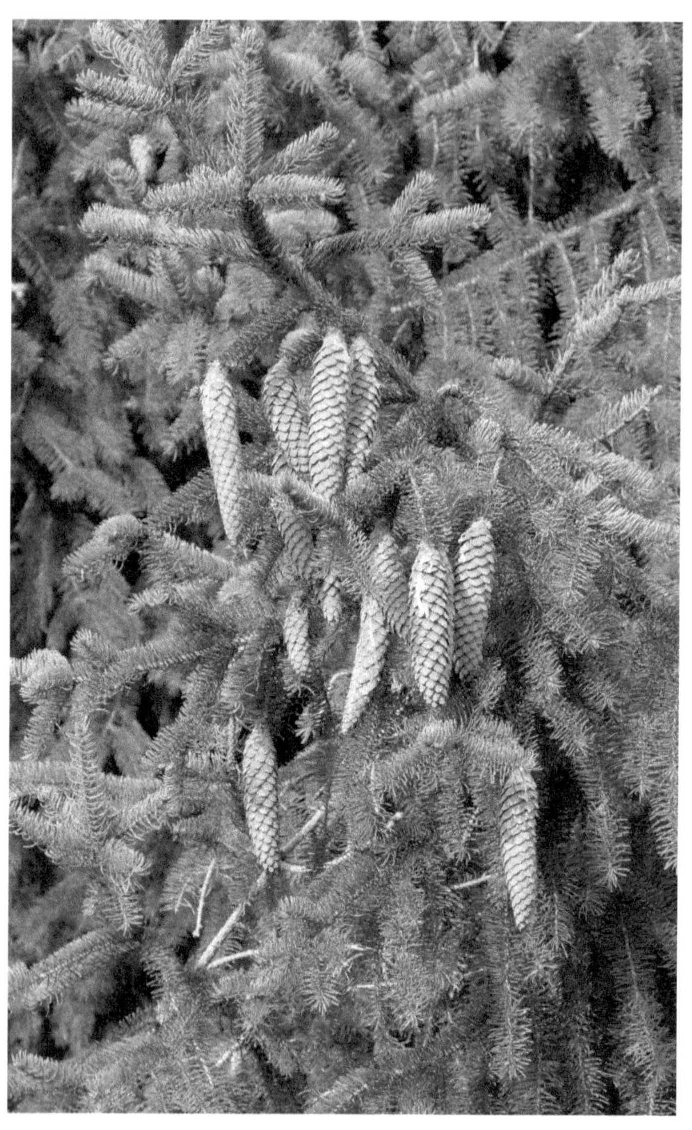

common spruce

The *red beech* (Latin: Fagus sylvatica) is a deciduous tree native in many parts of Europe. It is the only kind of beech native in central Europe so is there called simply the beech.

In Germany, it makes up about 15% of the deciduous trees in woodland. It is known as the *red beech* owing to the reddish hue of its wood, which is used for various items such as furniture.

The *red beech* is green in summer and can last for up to 300 years or occasionally even more. Mostly it reaches a height of up to 30m, but in longing for the sun in dense woodland, it may even reach a height of 45 m.

In Germany, the *red beech* was the tree of the year in 1990.

The beech stands for energy and strength, as well as for wisdom, clarity, shelter and durability. It implies that life should be relished here and now. The beech especially favors spiritual activity and efforts to overcome narrow-mindedness. It also offers patience and perseverance.

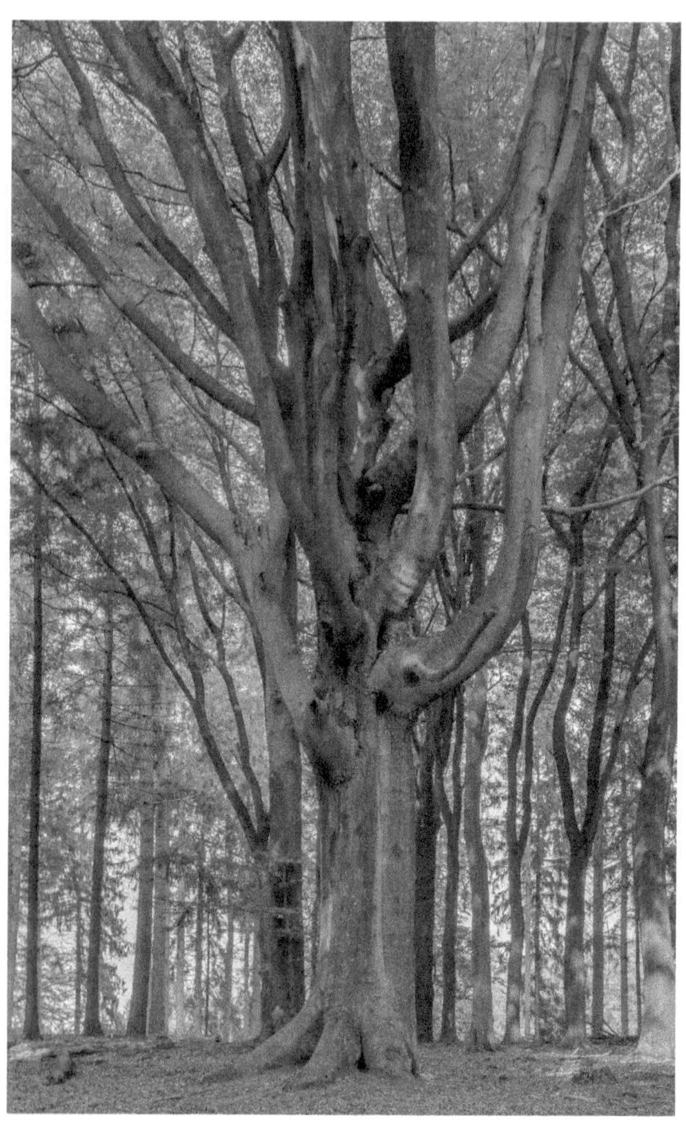

© depositphotos - Catstyecam

beech

The *Scots pine* (Latin: Pinus sylvestris), also known as the *Riga pine*, *Norway pine* and *Mongolian pine* is found from Europe to Siberia. After the *common spruce*, it is the most common tree in German woodland, where it is found on 22.9% of the area, but for several decades, the conversion of woods from mono-cultures to mixed cultures has also bee affecting pure pinewoods. The Scots pine is a fast-growing, evergreen conifer able to reach a height of 48 m and to live for 600 years.

For reasons of forestry and the timber industry, the *Scots pine* is one of the trees most often planted in Germany. It is uncommonly robust and easily looked after and supplies a lot of usable wood under even unfavorable conditions. The soil may be dry and poor in nutrients, but the tree remains undeterred.

The *Scots pine* supplies timber for buildings, furniture and floorboards.

Essential oil from its needles is used in medicine as well as in liniments and salves.

The *Scots pine* was the tree of the year in Germany in 2007

It is a symbol of long life, resilience and modesty. Two pines close together stand for love and faithfulness in marriage.

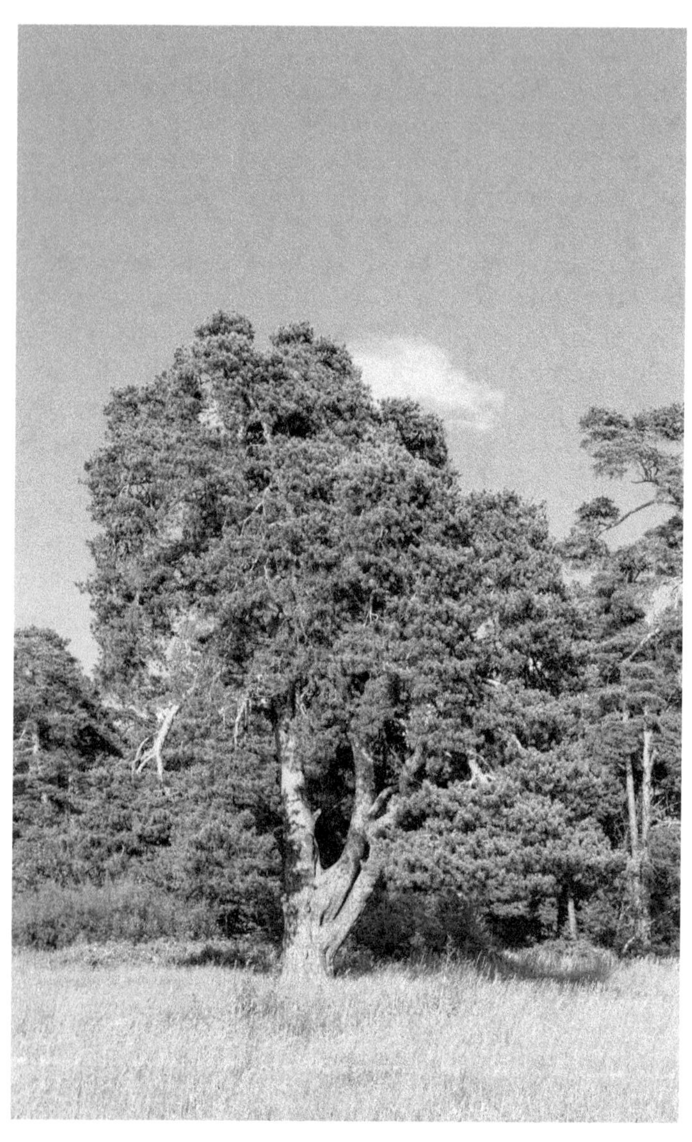

© depositphotos - Alx Yago

old scotch pine

Oak

In Germany, *oaks* make up about 11.5% of woodland, where they are the second most common kind of deciduous tree after *red beeches*.

The main kinds are the *common oak* (Latin: Quercus robur), also known as the *pedunculate, European* or *English oak*, and the *sessile oak* (Latin: Quercus petraea), also known as the *Cornish* or *durmast oak*. They are known respectively in Germany as the *summer oak* and the *winter oak*, perhaps because the former is found mainly in warm lowlands and the latter in cooler uplands. Both are called *white oaks* in German.

The *common oak* grows to a height of 20 to 40 m and may live for up to 500 or even 1000 years. In exceptional cases, they may grow to be 1 400 years old.

Oaks grow slowly and are sometimes, though seldom, found in the form of bushes.

In Germany, the *common oak* was the tree of the year in 1989, and the sessile oak in 2014.

An unusual feature of an *oak* is that it may harbor up to 1000 kinds of insects in its crown.

Its wood is used to make very valuable furniture and floorboards. Owing to a lot of tannin in it, the wood is very resistant and can be stored a long time.

Its bark was formerly used in the field of medicine for various purposes but is no longer.

The *oak* is known widely as the *'queen of the woods'*.

Since *oaks* are strong and long-lasting, they symbolize longevity and eternity. They stand for honesty, virtue and truth and for freedom, conviction and determination.

The *oak* was widely viewed as a holy, so no one was allowed to fell one.

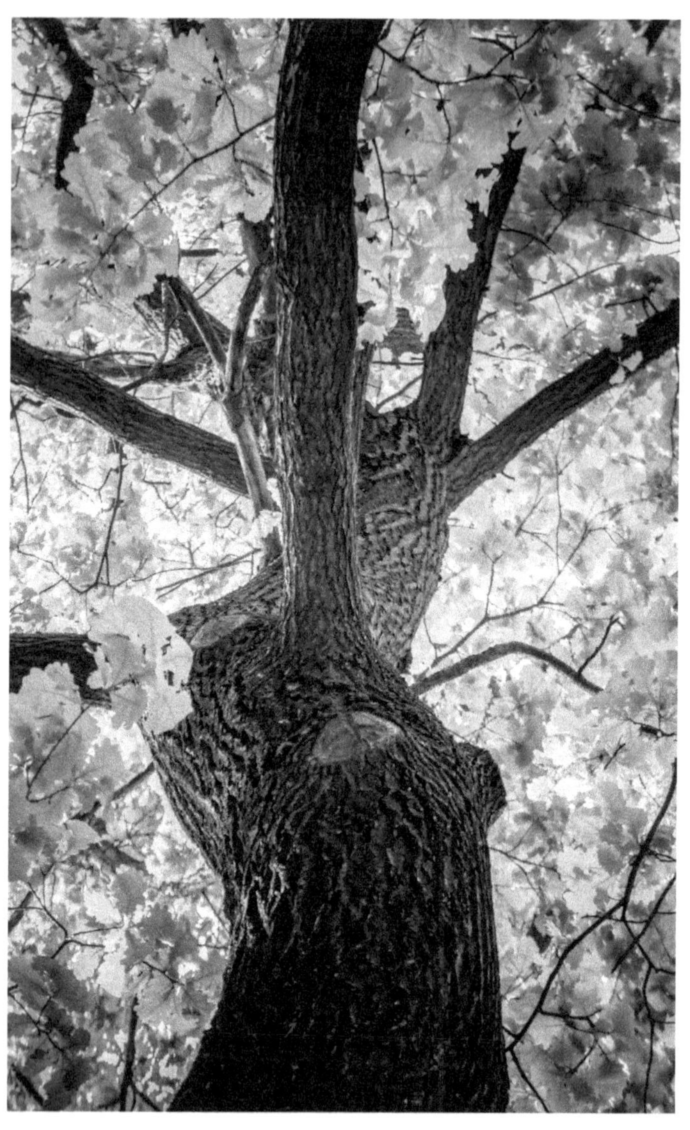

© depositphotos - gilmanshin

german oak

The *silver fir* (Latin: Abies alba) is a European conifer from the family of *pine trees* (Latin: Pinaceae). The tree's name is due to its light grey bark.

The *silver fir* can live for 500 or 600 years and reach a height of 30 to 50 m or occasionally 65 m.

The number of *silver firs* has fallen sharply for various reasons over the last 200 years. For one thing, it is the native tree most vulnerable to pests so has been decimated by many invasive kinds like the silver fir louse, besides having its leaves eaten by fallow and red deer. The number has also been lessened by clear-cut and over-use. In Germany, it now makes up only 1.7% of woodland.

Wood from the *silver fir* is used mainly for furniture, windows, doors and floorboards.

The *silver fir* was the tree of the year in Germany in 2004.

It is a symbol of beauty, strength and size, and firs in general stand for the triumph of light over darkness.

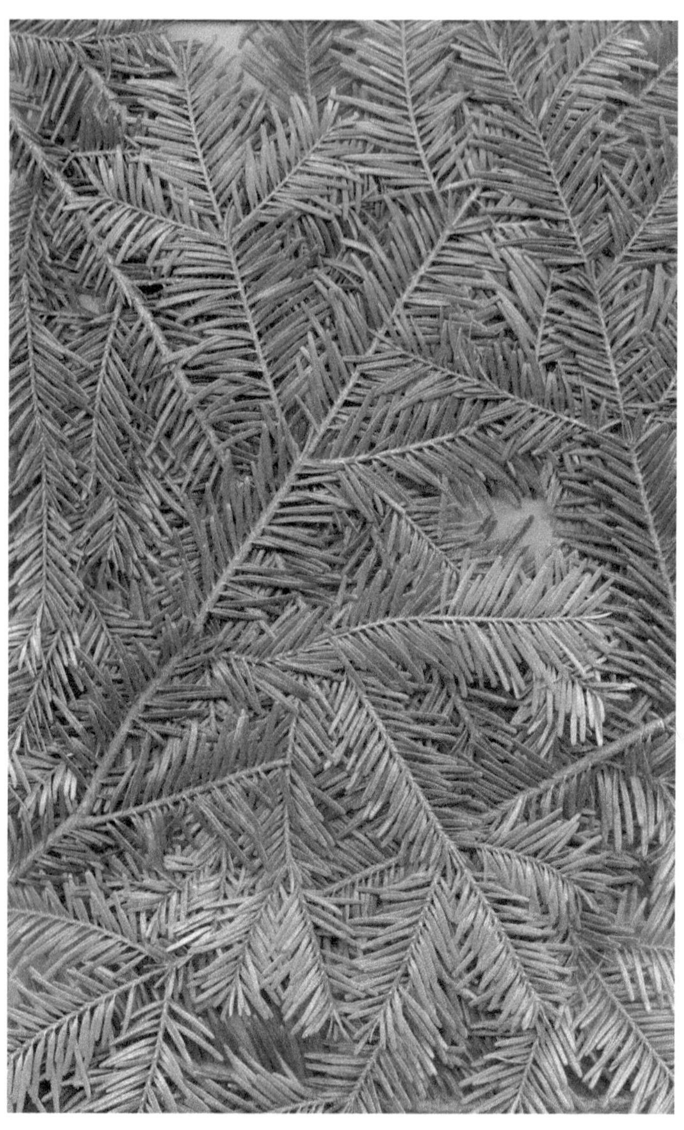

© depositphotos - ManfredKoch

branches of the silver fir

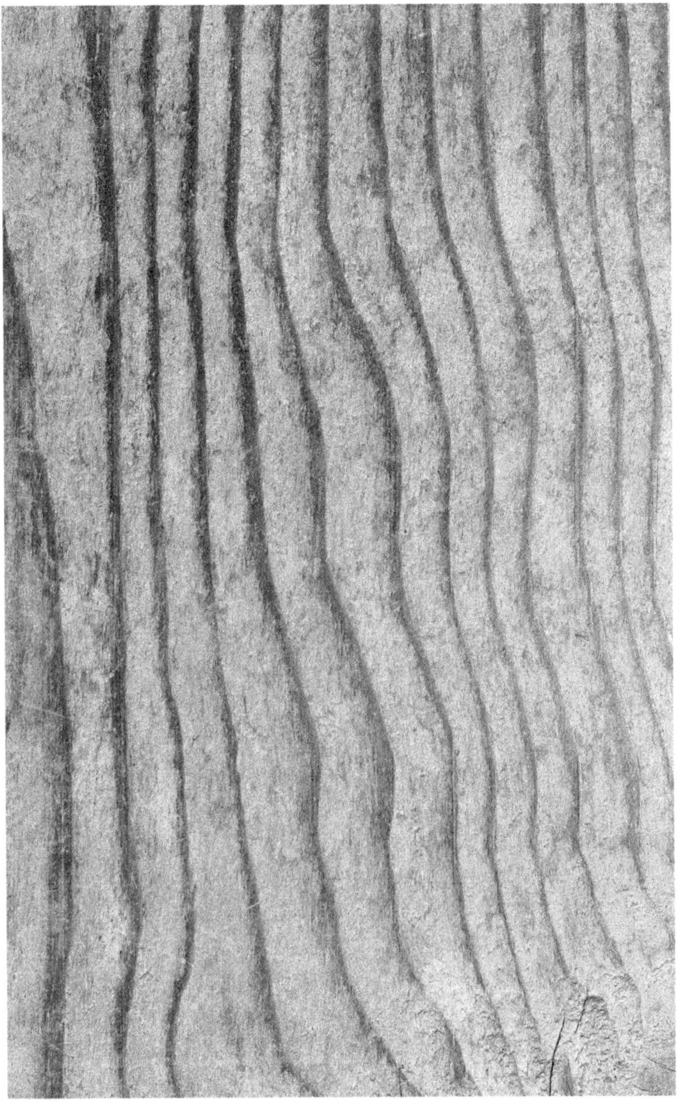

© depositphotos - taviphoto

silver fir bark texture

The *silver birch* (Latin: Betula pendula), otherwise called the *warty birch*, *European white birch*, or *East Asian white birch*, belongs to the family of birches. It is native to central and northern Europe and grows in southern Europe only in mountainous regions. It is a pioneer tree in being one of the first to settle in fallow areas, and in being swift to grow, it is the epitome of youth and lives no longer than 160 years.

The *silver birch* also has an eminent role in folklore. It was revered as holy long before the oak and linden. At this time the custom began of cutting a tree in the woodland down as a maypole. It was a way to bring spring and nature into a village and is still familiar today in many places.

The *silver birch* is the epitome of spring, of new ventures and reawakening life. It stands for vitality and the removal of toxins and poisons from parts of a body, rejuvenating it as a whole.

Leaves from the *silver birch* may be used for making teas, juices or elixirs for healing purposes, as the body is thereby cleansed and detoxified. Slags, acids and other substances burdening and weakening the body are rinsed away, and the kidneys are activated. In general, the silver birch stands for processes related to this flow and renewal. Owing to its vitalizing effect, exhaustion and weakness are soon alleviated. Oil from the *silver birch* can also be applied externally to remove waste products and to strengthen the body. The good qualities of the leaves are due mainly to flavonoids but also to volatile oils, saponins, tannins, bitter substances and vitamin C. The leaves can most easily be used to make tea. Even the elixir, made by gently cooking the young leaves and preserving them with sugar, is suitable for curative application.

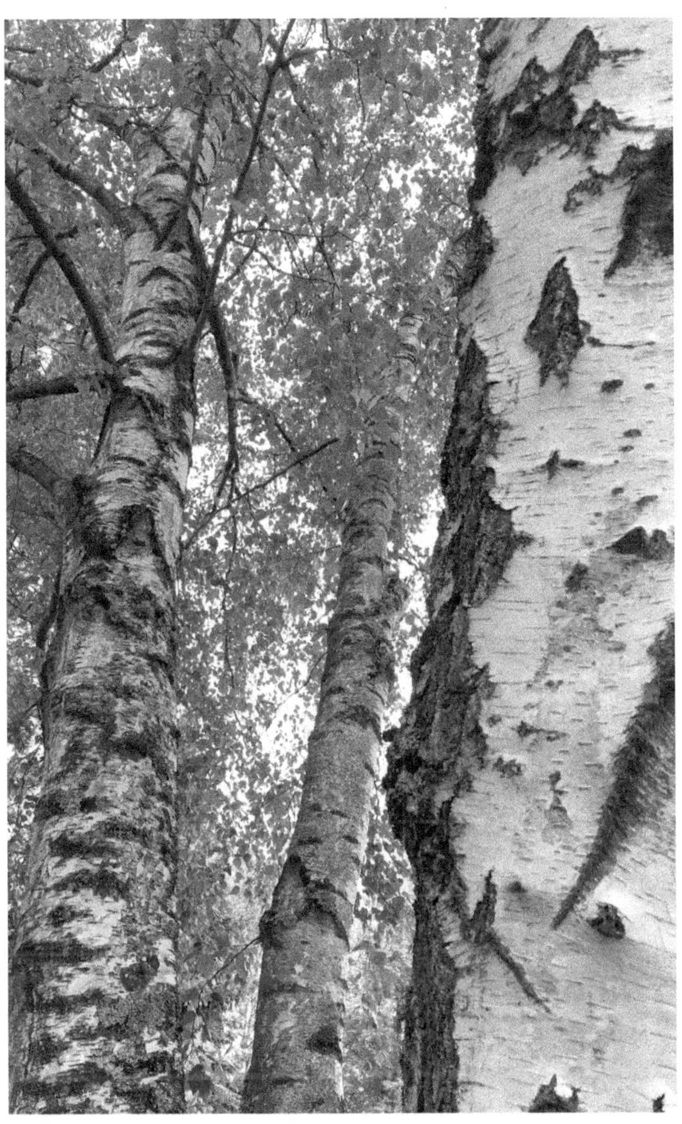

© depositphotos - studiograndouest

silver birch

There would be no life without woodland

Before there were woods, there was so little oxygen in the air that life as we know it could hardly exist. Only when trees made up for this lack did life as we know it begin. This is why a wood is often known as a green lung, since the green hue is due to the presence of chlorophyll, which converts lots of carbon dioxide into oxygen, important for life.

Woodland, however, does much more for the landscape and climate, as well as supplying us with useful materials. Its importance as an ecosystem can hardly be exaggerated.

In what other ways we are greatly supported by woodland is detailed below.

Woodland stores and purifies

One of the most important services rendered by woodland is the storage and purification of water.

Rain or snow do not remain on the surface and flow away but are mainly sponged up by the soil. This can take huge amounts of water in, so it offers excellent protection against flooding. At the same time, woodland filters and purifies water, and the resulting pure water is rich in oxygen and excellent for drinking.

More positive effects of woodland will be detailed later.

Woodland protects from erosion

Woodland protects soil from erosion by holding it in place by its webs of roots. Moreover, the crowns and umbrellas of leaves slow any rain down, lessening its ability to wash soil away.

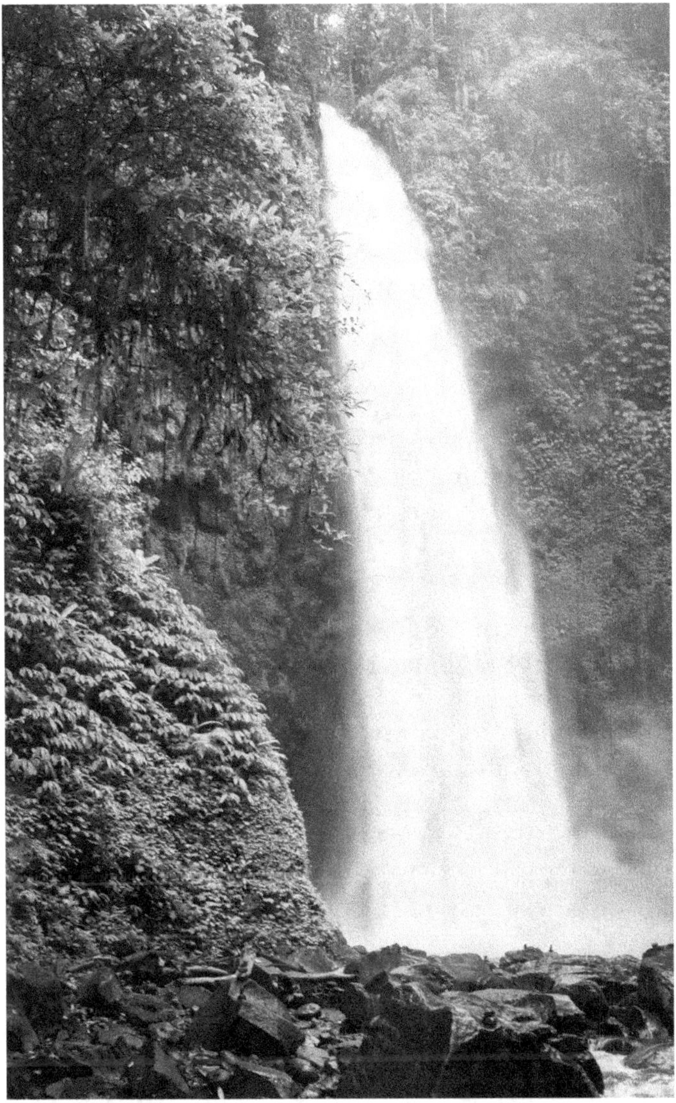

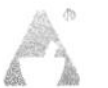

© depositphotos - Keola

waterfall at woodland

Woodland protects from avalanches

In regions with steep inclines, woodland is a key protection against avalanches, as its trees hold a good portion back.

Woodland binds pollutants

Its leaves filter out dust and gaseous pollutants, so woodland is also important in purifying the air.

Woodland contributes to climate protection

Woodland lessens daily and yearly fluctuations in temperature and increases humidity and condensation. Big connected stretches of woodland near urban areas improve their climate.

Woodland as a source of wood

Wood is one of the few renewable and environmentally friendly raw materials available to us. A sustainable timber industry, in which fewer trees are felled than are allowed to grow has by now become a reality in Germany, though woodland is still being wantonly destroyed on a huge scale in some other countries, especially in the tropics.

Woodland as a habitat

Compared to other biotopes, woodland has an immense variety of flora, fauna and fungi, many of which have adapted specifically to this environment. It often serves as the last refuge for shy animals, who are unable to fare well in more populated areas.

Woodland as a leisure area

Woodland, especially within reach of town-dwellers, is important for leisure. The mild climate, tranquility and variety of impressions refresh and revitalize many visitors.

Woodland and the soul, spirit and body

Being in woodland is like bathing in summer. All facets of our lives benefit from the pleasure in many ways.

There are many reasons why dalliance in woodland is uniquely good for the health. Not only is there the play of light and shade and the tang of scents but also the tranquility, as sounds are muted by leaves and loam. The effects are not only additive but also synergetic, enhancing each other.

We instinctively feel the benefit of being there. Soul and spirit are calmed and refreshed, and the world outside can no longer impose stress. Moreover, we spend much of our time in woodland moving around, which has all-round benefits for the otherwise sedentary.

Woodland stands for restfulness, relaxation, focus, equanimity, power and healing, but it not only stands for these qualities, it also induces them in us.

Dalliance in woodland is like having a brief holiday or health cure. We return to everyday life with new reserves of energy and strength and feeling years younger.

Just how wonderfully woodland enhances our health will be detailed below.

The special atmosphere of woodland affects especially the way we feel. Even a few minutes in the midst of greenery are often enough to dissipate our daily vexation and care. In reaction to the calmness around us, our bodies too calm down with the help of the parasympathetic nervous system. This dilutes the concentrations of the stress hormones cortisol and adrenaline, while increasing the concentrations of happiness hormones like serotonin and dopamine.

Consequently, inner unrest, anxiety, aggression and depression are toned down or eliminated, and grudges and obsessions yield to love of life and to spells of happiness.

Visiting woodland swiftly reduces stress. Owing to the many beneficial natural impressions, agitation is calmed and soothed. A feeling of peace, rest and harmony pervade our being, and our nerves become less touchy. In woodland, our perception of the world is enriched and has a chance to become less gloomy.

Woodland, attention and equanimity

By heeding everything happening in woodland, we become more attentive and even-tempered. Without hastening to pass judgment, we remain open to sights, sounds and scents. We dally in the here and now, enchanted by the flora and fauna. Nothing distracts us, and everyday life fades in the distance. Feelings of ease and gratitude enhance our inner peace and gain the upper hand.

While dallying in woodland, we put everyday cares aside and empty our minds, which are then free to heed other things. It may sound paradoxical that emptying our minds somehow improves them but this is not very mysterious. In everyday life, we have to pay attention to many different things at the same time, so we find it very hard to focus.

In woodland, we are no less attentive but also relaxed. We are no longer entangled in our thoughts and concerns but are open to fresh inspiration and new impressions. We may focus on something as simple as a trunk, a branch, a twig or a leaf, incidentally strengthening our powers of concentration, our ability to learn from new impressions and to play with them creatively.

Even memory is exercised and the process of aging slowed down. Our thoughts and feelings become clearer and we become more inquisitive and inspired.

Those of us often troubled by respiratory ailments such as bronchitis, inflammation of the nasal cavities, runny noses and colds in general should visit woodland regularly. Even chronically obstructive ailments of the lungs like COPD or tuberculosis can be eased by strolling there. This is due mainly to essential oils lavishly bestowed by the needles, tips of twigs and branches of spruces, firs and pines, which loosen slime, disinfect the airways and lessen inflammation. These keep ailments of the respiratory organs in check.

Moreover, the fresh, unpolluted air is purifying and liberating. The greater humidity is a boon for dry airways, as moisture hinders the passage of bacteria, viruses and dust.

A slight warning is needed only by people allergic to pollen, who should seasonally refrain from going on long hikes there.

Woodland helps the blood circulate

Wandering through woodland strengthens the circulatory system, lowers high blood pressure and slows a frenetic pulse. These effects are due partly to movement but also to the fact that the vegetative nervous system switches over into its restful mode, lessening concentrations of the stress hormones cortisol and adrenalin. This in turn lowers the blood pressure and relieves the circulatory system, while stimulating production of the hormone DHEA (dehydroepiandrosterone), to protect the system.

Woodland stimulates the immune system

When we wander through woodland, the combination of moving, breathing fresh terpenes in and the whole stress-free ambiance strengthens and stimulates the immune system. Stress hormones such as cortisol and adrenaline are lessened, thereby stabilizing the system indirectly.

As pointed out above, terpenes also increase the number of killer cells in the blood by 40% and their activity by 50%. Killer cells in turn increase the body's powers of resistance in belonging to the nonspecific part of the immune system.

There is also evidence of an increase in the production of anti-cancer proteins, which help killer cells deal with any cancerous cells encountered.

Woodland keeps us limber

Wandering in woodland lubricates the joints and benefits the whole musculoskeletal system. Especially today, when many people suffer from lack of movement, wandering in woodland is a fine way to let stiff and underused joints get back on form without undue stress. It is especially useful if we have not indulged in sport for a long time and wish to get back on form. The wandering exercises all our muscles, including those of the legs and back. Regions round the rump are strengthened, the spine is relaxed and the body as a whole becomes more flexible. Whoever has chronic pains of the joints or back soon feels an improvement. Our feet too are exercised in woodland. The loam surface is a blessing for our soles, especially if we walk barefoot for awhile. The foot reflex zones are massaged, benefiting the whole body.

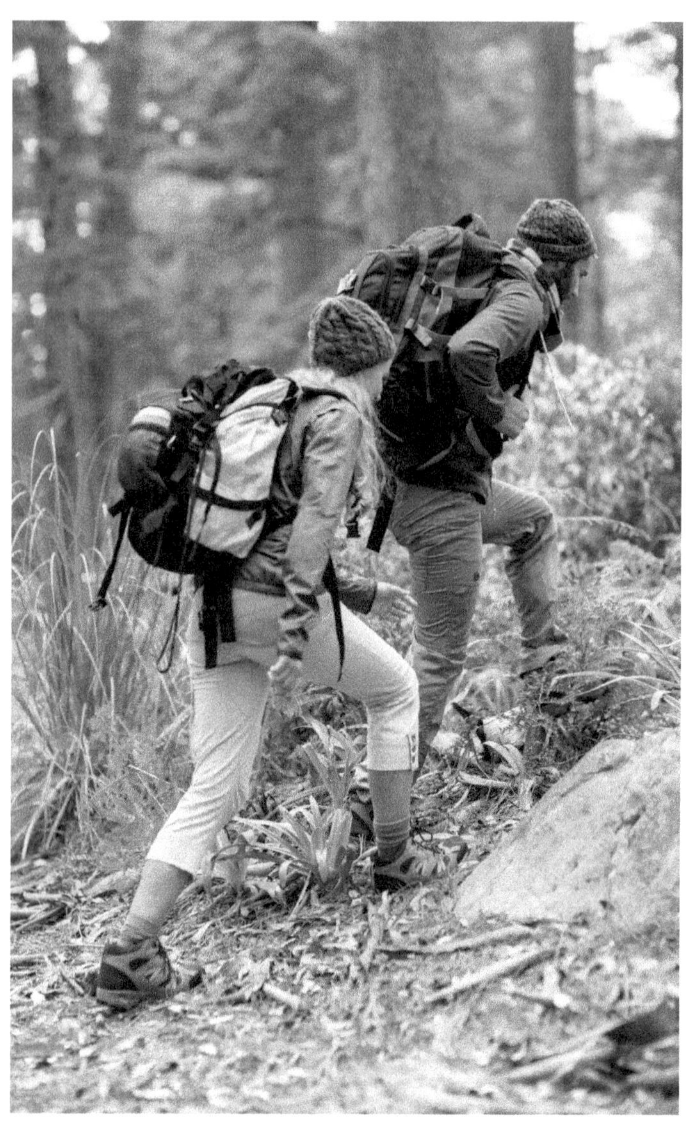

© depositphotos - Wavebreakmedia

hike at woodland

The fresh air and the mild clime of woodland ease or banish headaches. Whoever suffers continually from headaches should not hesitate to wander through woodland as a useful treatment without any bad side effects.

Woodland helps us to sleep soundly

Whether we are likely to sleep soundly depends less on our bedtime habits than on how we have spent the day.

If the day has been pleasant, our dreams tend to be so too. After all, while asleep, we process the events of the day, so their nature is bound to influence the quality of our sleep. If our days are restless and anxious or we are stressed from all sides, we do not go to bed alone but take with us our grudges and grievances.

Hence, if we avoid stress as much as possible during the day, we have less to avoid at night, and there is hardly a better way to avoid stress than to wander through woodland. Benign hours without stress in the greenery together with the fresh air and movement are the best preconditions for a healthy and regenerative sleep.

Plants' personalities

Just as every plant grows differently to other similar plants, and just as leaves and petals spread different scents, and the fruit of one plant tastes different to that of another, all plants have their own typical qualities.

You may have noticed somewhere that a tree or a photo of a tree seems to have a face growing out of the trunk. Was it, perhaps, a sign of the tree's nature? Wander with open eyes through woodland and you may notice some plants or trees, which capture your attention through their unusual growth or other peculiarities.

Plants' personalities, their individual traits and powers were preoccupations of some women in the Middle Ages, who were known as herbal witches. Likewise, the shamans of many peoples, natural healers, homeopaths and modern practitioners of the esoteric have viewed plants as individuals. They have used them for healing purposes but also for incense. *Druids*, the so-called tree-spirits, knew how to communicate with trees and plants and made strong drinks from them, each of which had a specific use.

The word *druid* came originally from *dru-wid*, though it is still an open question as to whether dru stood for an oak as such or for a wood as a gateway to another world, whereas wid meant wise. In other words, druids were wise people with insight into the nature of trees and woodland.

In homeopathy and Bach flower therapy, the essences of plants are used for transferring the plants' qualities and powers to the people treated or to induce in them the same vibrations. This transference of force and energy from the plants is meant to stimulate the self-healing powers of the body, to restore its natural and healthy equilibrium.

Even the burning of plants as incense is meant to free their essence, which can then be sensed and effective on a subtler level.

These are all examples of how we may interact with the powers and personalities of plants.

Plants' souls

Since time immemorial, certain qualities have been attributed to plants, as shown by many cultures and myths. Not only the *alphabet of runes* but also the Celtic alphabet of trees, *Ogham*, has its place in the domain of plants. These alphabets are by no means like the alphabet beginning with a, b and c, since every letter in them is also a symbol, which together with its sound is associated with a certain force of nature. Since these forces flow through all things, these alphabets are also an expression of plants' souls.

In some cultures, trees and plants have been integrated into human life, according to the spiritual powers attributed to them. For instance, there was the thing-tree, under which verdicts were passed and important assemblies were held. The thing-tree was mostly an oak or linden but could also be the oldest tree in a village, as this was taken to be the wisest. A thing-square was often surrounded by seven lindens, and lindens were said to have prophetic and healing qualities. The Celts even had a tree-horoscope, and a tree's soul was taken to be linked with everyone born under its sign.

The oak was the holy tree of the druids and in some Celtic traditions was associated with Thor, the god of thunder. It was said to have magical powers and to offer protection. The ash, or sometimes the yew, was the tree where Odin was said to have been initiated. Odin was the foremost god in Norse mythology and was held to be the gods' father and the god of death but also of poetry and runes, magic and ecstasy. Thor, the god of thunder, was nonetheless widely revered.

From Genesis in the Bible, we are familiar with the tree of knowledge of good and evil (Latin: lignum sapientae boni et mali), which grew in the middle of the garden of Eden or paradise by the the tree of life and whose fruit was taboo. A further remnant of old beliefs and heathen culture is the Christmas tree decked with candles, to mark the winter solstice and the sun-god's resurrection.

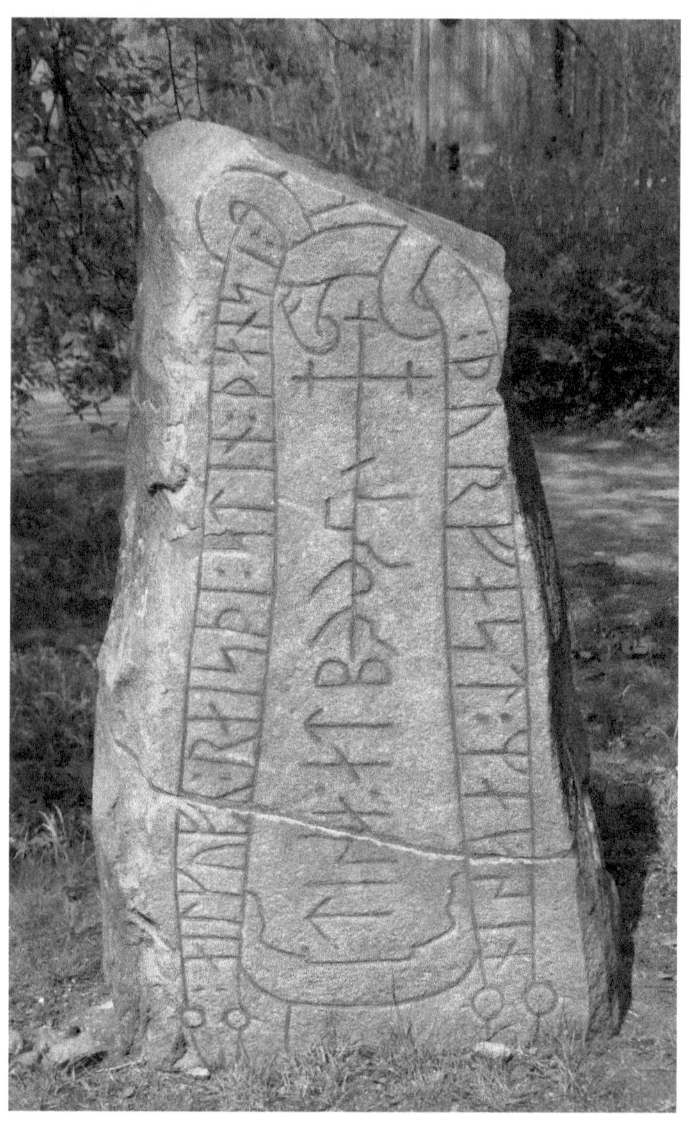

© depositphotos - mylips

antique runestone

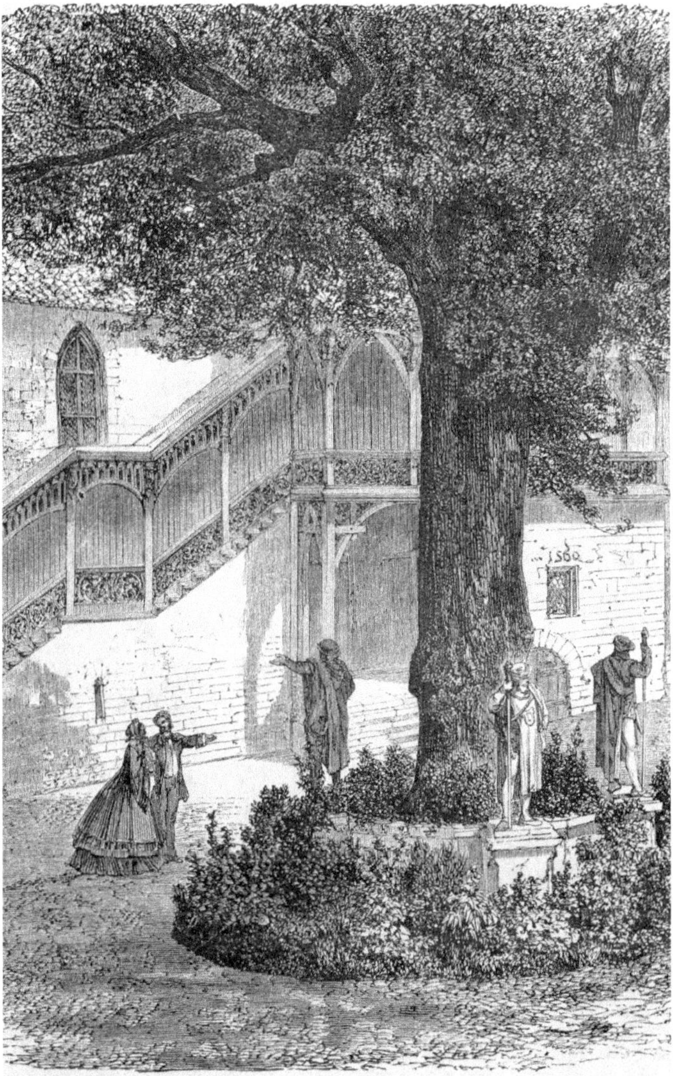

© depositphotos - marzolino

court tree old linden

The above examples show the traditional interest in trees and their hidden powers.

Every kind of tree was said to have its own nature. If a grove was made up of only one kind of tree, it was said to be especially holy, as the powers of the separate trees all added up. There were various kinds of groves such as fertility groves and groves for divination or shelter.

There were not only separate kinds of trees, each with its own nature, but also spirits, whose fates were bound up with the trees. If a tree died, so did its spirit. Further essences of trees were known as nymphs, also linked to waters or mountains. In effect, some of the nymphs were thought to be inseparable from trees, whereas others could move around freely as if thoughts sent out by the trees.

In Greek and Roman mythology, nymphs were female nature spirits, and those living in trees were known as dryads, a word relating them to the druids. The tree nymphs could be understood as trees' protectors and higher selves like the higher selves of humans. Whether bound to a tree or free to move around, they were beings with whom the initiated came into contact and whose powers they were able to use through ceremonies and rituals.

In Greek mythology, a dryad was originally only a nymph of an oak, as shown for instance by the fact that the word for an oak in Greek was dys, but the word dryad was later used for tree-nymphs in general.

A dryad was thought to be closely linked to the tree she lived in and to be able to change her appearance to match the tree's. She was an especially important and beautiful kind of nymph. Even today, we can get in touch with these nature spirits of plants and trees and ask for their protection, while revering and protecting them ourselves.

If a leaf falls from a tree, part of the tree's power and specific energy is still in the leaf, and the same was thought to be true of a tree-spirit. Only when a leaf withers or decays or is burned as incense, is this energy dissipated and transformed. Hence, the gifts of a tree are valuable, as we are able to use the powers present in them and to appreciate them as gestures of friendship.

Many of the powers present in trees can be divined. We can watch their crowns swaying in the wind and see that they do not merely yield. Rather, if they are grouped together as in woodland, some sway in one direction and others in others, thereby lessening the force of the wind and the likelihood of damage. The wind has only to fell one big tree for this to fell others, but if its force is stemmed, even frailer trees are able to survive. Trees' motion in wind is determined mainly by the trees themselves, who behave elastically and flexibly instead of merely yielding.

Their lesson for us is that we should place both feet firmly on the ground, as if rooted, not letting ourselves be felled by strokes of adversity. We need to feel certain of ourselves but also to be flexible, then we are able to survive unharmed in even turbulent times.

As already mentioned, trees can also use protective and defense mechanisms and, if threatened, may warn other trees nearby, who in turn warn more.

Trees thereby help each other if nutrients are scarce and can strategically react in many ways to changes in their surroundings. If infected by harmful bacteria, they produce antibiotics, which stimulate even the human immune system.

Our forebears, whose lives were much closer to nature than ours, observed trees' reactions and drew conclusions about their qualities and powers. If in doubt, they relied on the advice of wise men and women, who were able to communicate with trees and their nature spirits. Trees were viewed as protective beings, ensuring the continuity of life.

They were a link between above and below, between the world of the gods and the world of mankind, so runes and the letters of the Celtic ogham alphabet were originally made up of twigs. According to the kind of tree and its characteristics, the powers latent within it were thought to differ. People were aware of the qualities of each kind of plant and of their possible use for healing or other purposes.

We may drink even today from this pool of knowledge, or we can look at plants and trees for ourselves and draw our own conclusions.

In many places it is still customary to plant a tree at the birth of a child or on settling down in a new home, and the custom is also found in myths. People sought the protection of a tree with a tree-spirit, whose support they wished to be granted.

Trees were also planted for other purposes. Gifts were offered to them and their spirits, to secure their favors. This applied not only to tree-spirits but also to other nature-spirits using the trees as homes.

Woodland, with trees towering up and forming a green canopy, were felt to be holy. The domes of cathedrals with their pillars may have been based on this experience.

In strolling on paths among trees, people felt the tranquility to be a divine source of vitality. The rustling and whispering of the crowns seemed to be recalling past events and to be presaging events to come, and people also sought healing or solutions to their problems in groves.

Totems were made from the wood of certain trees, to create cult sites. Gatherings of trees as woods or groves were oracular places, linking various worlds and serving as the homes of fairies and elves.

Every tree was like the world-tree in linking seen and unseen dimensions, microcosm and macrocosm, past and future, so every tree had a part to play in the ensemble, according to its own nature.

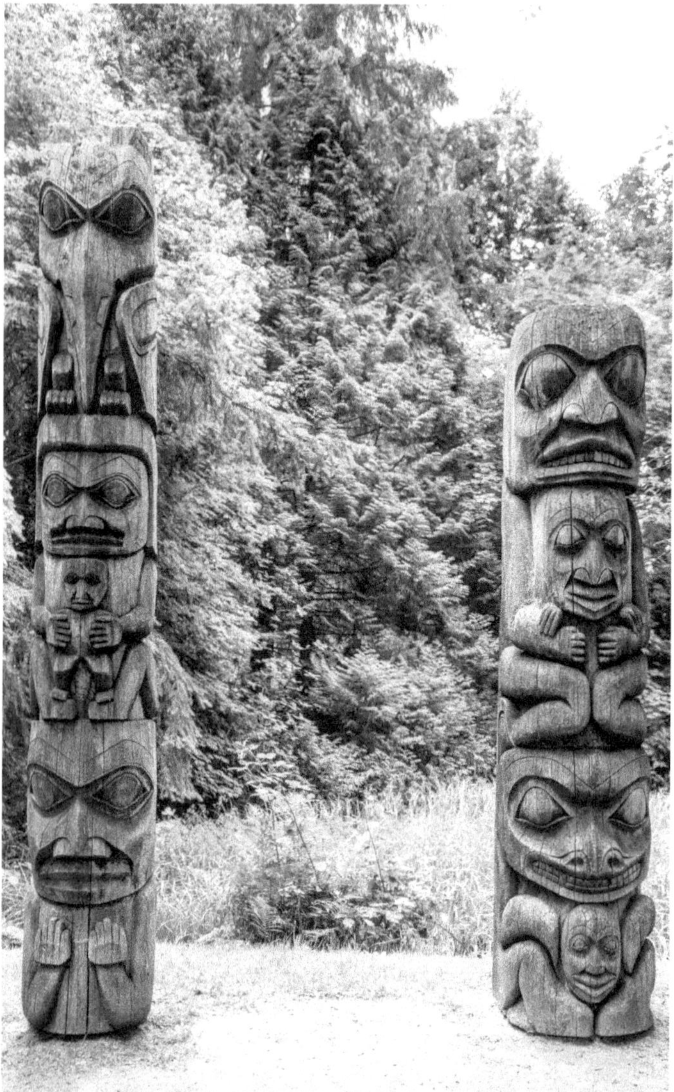

© depositphotos - dbvirago

totem poles

The world-tree

This stands in many cultures for the whole cosmos with its various planes and dimensions in being the pillar of the world, the tree of life and the bearer of all worlds. Among the Celts it was known as the Yggdrasil, among the Germans as Irminsul, the pillar of the earth and the midpoint of many worlds.

The trunk of the world-trees links heaven and earth; its roots reach deep into the underworld; its upper branches soar into the heavens and other ethereal realms; and its lower branches reach into the world of everyday.

Much the same is true of the world-tree in the cabbala, whose sephiroth stand for various dimensions and transitions into other worlds.

The astral world is the world of souls. There is a world inhabited by the dead or forebears, also a world of the gods, the personified basic powers, and finally there is an underworld as their source.

All these and other worlds are linked by the world-tree.

In kundalini yoga, a person is taken to be an earthly version of the world-tree or a miniature version of the cosmos. Everything is linked to everything else, and we are parts of the whole.

Kundalini-yoga is a kind of yoga meant to increase a person's vitality. It works on the astral body and its chakras, which are centers of energy, and on nadis, which are channels of energy. The yoga exercises are meant to cleanse the astral body and to harmonize the chakras.

In kundalini-yoga, the energy flows through a person's spine like sap through the trunk of a tree. Just as a trunk splits up into branches and these into twigs, the ethereal channels of energy in a person likewise divide and subdivide into the nadis.

The chakras are vortexes of energy and offer us access to higher planes of experience. Kundalini is a serpentine power or pure vitality, which rises from the realm of the earth and moves upward toward the divine. It flows through the spine, linking the planes, from the lower to the higher, like sap in the world-tree.

Like the world-tree linking this world with other worlds, the spine thereby links all the facets of life and the powers of nature, as do the trunks of other trees. We can judge the character and qualities of trees by their outer appearance, not only in the sense of the visible but also in the sense of the fragrant or tangible, by rubbing a leaf, smelling a blossom or eating a fruit for instance. This material envelopes a living being, whose character and qualities are likewise specific to the tree.

In mythology, every tree is viewed as being a reflection of the world-tree, revealing the same principles of organization, though not all the original qualities. Different kinds of trees embody a different range of qualities, according to their nature, but their nature is not to be confused with a tree-spirit.

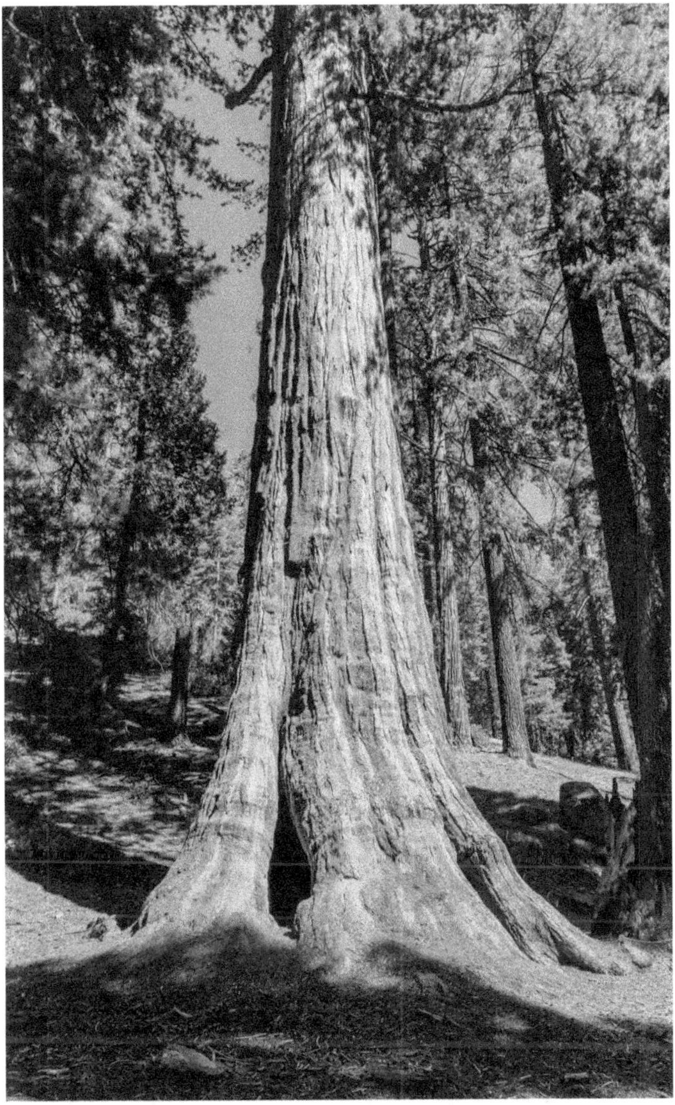

© depositphotos - durktalsma

sequoia between heaven and earth

Other trees and plants

In woodland, we are surrounded by many kinds of trees and plants, so it is hardly surprising that many of us like to stroll through woodland, admiring the rich variety. There were can replenish our reserves of energy, feel hidden and sheltered and experience a stroll as a process of purification. Woodland offers us a chance to withdraw from the rush and worry of everyday life and to regain our equilibrium in a tranquil atmosphere.

In woodland, we are improved in various ways by the interaction of many of the trees and plants around us, not to mention the scent of the moist earth and of the leaves and fruit. The play of light, as sunshine slants through the leafy crowns and the lofty trunks, lends us a feeling of sublimity and self-confidence.

Every separate tree and plant in woodland contributes to the overall impression and greatly affects our feelings, moods and vitality. According to our own natures and current situation in life, we address ourselves to one power or another. We feel most intensely whatever we need most and what resonates most deeply within us.

But of course, for this to take place, we have to open ourselves to woodland and the impressions which it is willing to make on us. Every tree and plant has a message of its own.

We can now take a closer look at the nature and magic of certain trees and plants, which we may happen to find in woodland.

This was the tree of the druids and stood for eternity and the cycle of growth and decay, of youth and age. In the Celtic Futhark, it tallied with the rune rhaido, the wheel of life.

Among the druids, the oak was also viewed as the gateway to a different world. Likewise, among shamans, the oak is the tree linking this world with the next.

According to mythology, the oak also offers protection from beings from other worlds such as demons, since it serves as a shut door, keeping them at bay.

If especially valuable, treasures were kept in oaken chests, and a front door of oak served to keep negative forces and ailments at bay.

The druids also valued oaks for the fact that they gathered mistletoe preferably from them for use in their magic and rituals.

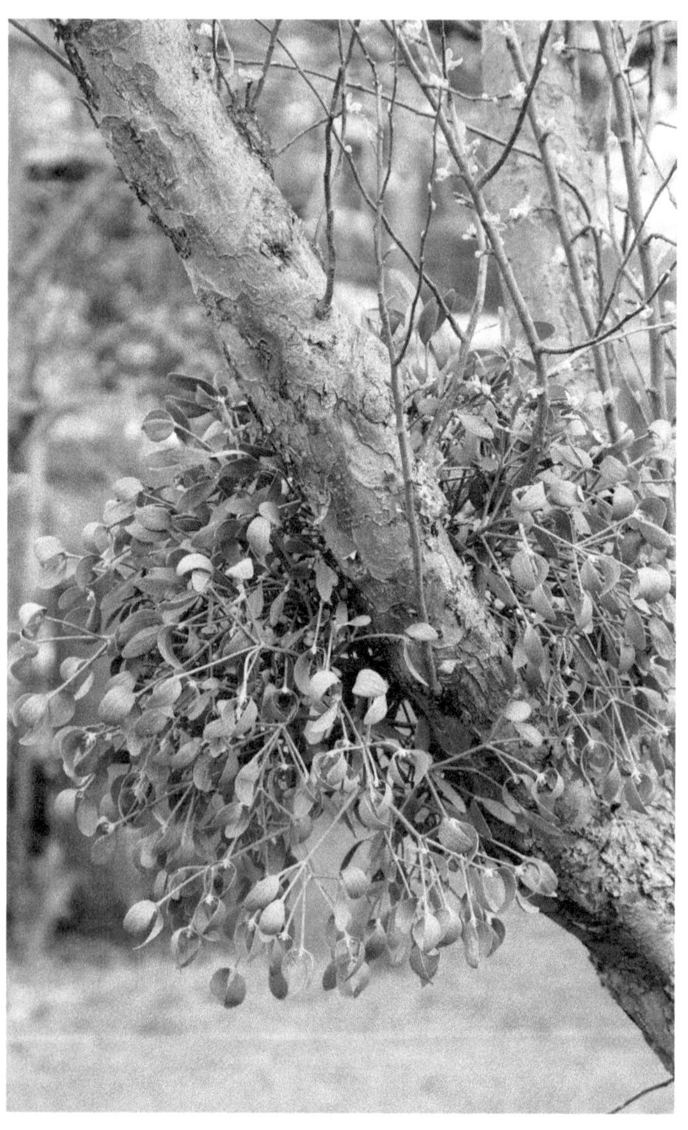

misteltoe

The willow prefers moist or swampy areas on the borders of woodland or on banks of nearby rivers and can mostly be recognized on account of its long and drooping twigs. There is something mystical about a willow, and at the same time its umbrella of leaves lends it an air of secrecy. In mythology, the door to the underworld is often revealed to be hidden beneath this canopy.

Notably, the willow has very pliant branches, which can be bent very much without breaking. This shows a high degree of flexibility as well as an ability to lean this way and that without basically changing position. The willow also has exceptional powers of regeneration, as twigs removed from it and left on the ground soon take root and begin growing, so the willow stands for healing and regeneration.

Hence the willow is ascribed to the rune laguz and to the moon of intuition. Its bark is a source of the pain-killer salicin, which also increases the circulation of the blood. In a processed and synthesized form (acetylsalicylic acid), it is also present in aspirin.

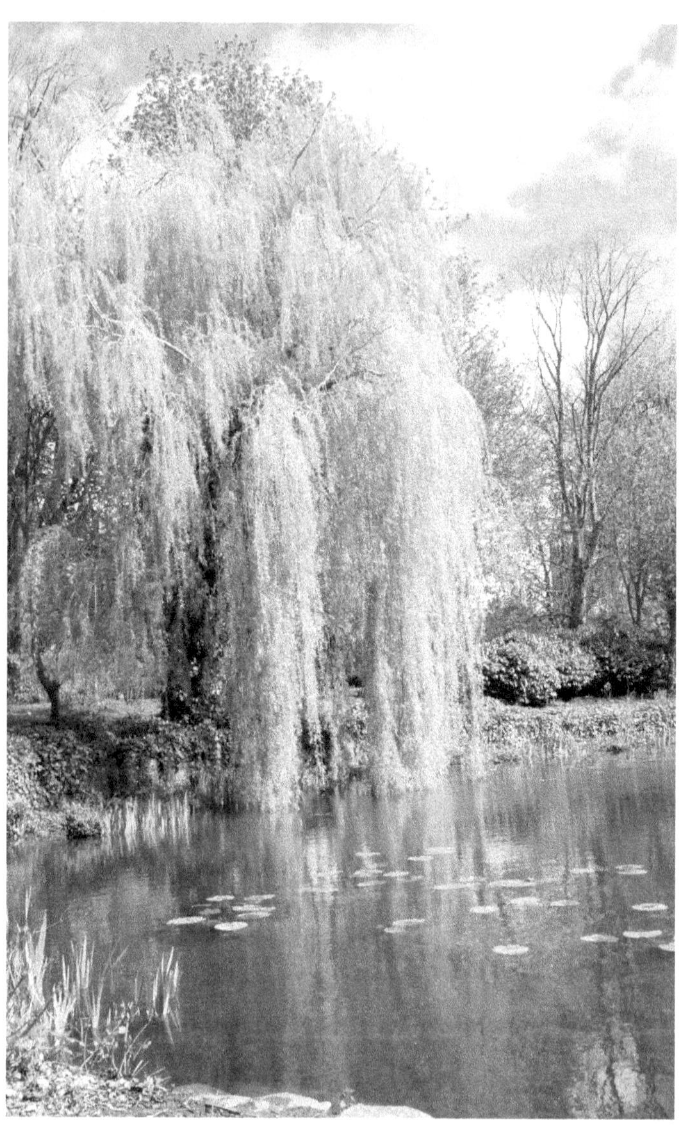

© depositphotos - pete776

Willow

Among the Celtic, the elderberry was said to offer an entrance to the underworld and access to the more ethereal world of the elves, fairies, dwarfs and domestic spirits. Elderberry twigs offered witches protection and a choice set of magical powers, so they were readily used as magic wands. In folklore, it is said that whoever has an elderberry tree in the garden or in front of the house can be sure of being protected by it, whereas whoever harms it is bound to suffer misfortune.

The elderberry stands for purification, a comprehensive view, insight and a connection to the world of forebears and natural spirits. It is represented by the rune hagalaz and the Germanic goddess Hel. The name of Mrs. Holle from the tale of the Brothers Grimm with the same name is likely to come from Hel, the name of the goddess of death.

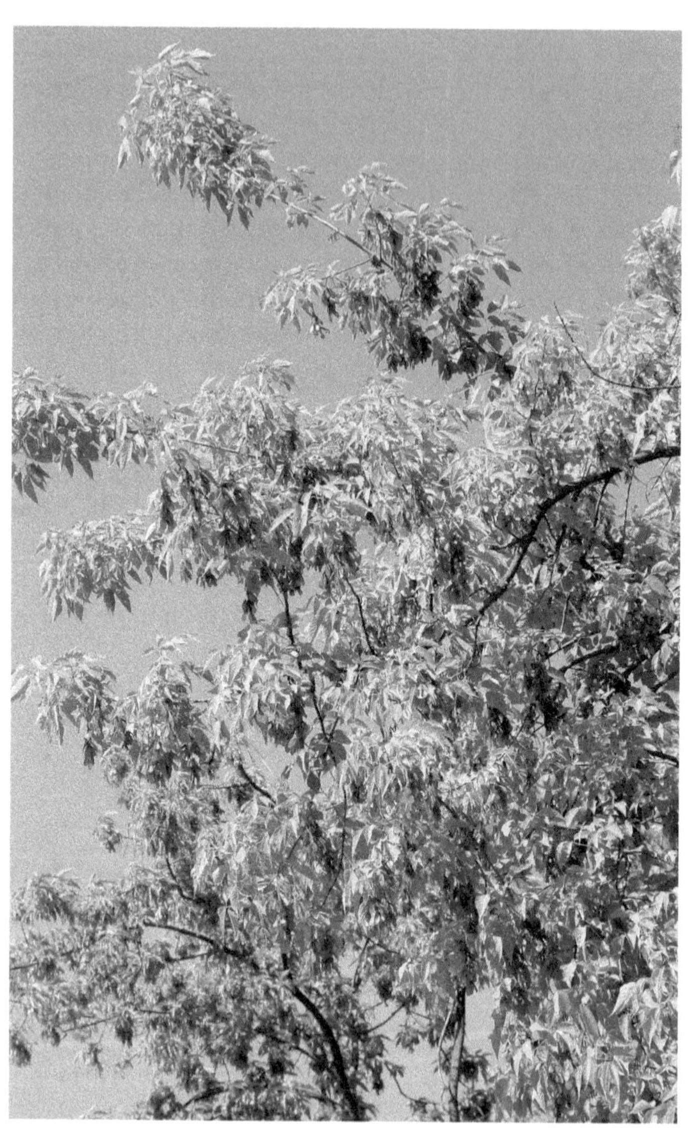

© depositphotos - Manka

Box elder with fruits

Among some peoples, the world-tree was said to be a common, European or English yew. In terms of mythology, it stands for everlasting life, magic and the power of forebears. The yew is also the tree under which Odin hung upside down for nine days and nights, to achieve knowledge. The yew leads us to the deepest levels of our own selves, lets us recognize our souls and opens our senses to other dimensions. If the druids wished to confer about something important or to gain the advice and support of higher powers, this was the tree they gathered under.

As an evergreen, the yew shows that it is strong enough to withstand the cycle of the year and to keep its leaves even in winter. With its poisonous needles, seeds and poisonous wood, it warns us to be careful in getting along with our own inner powers and also with the knowledge of the initiated, higher insights and the other-worldly powers of our forebears.

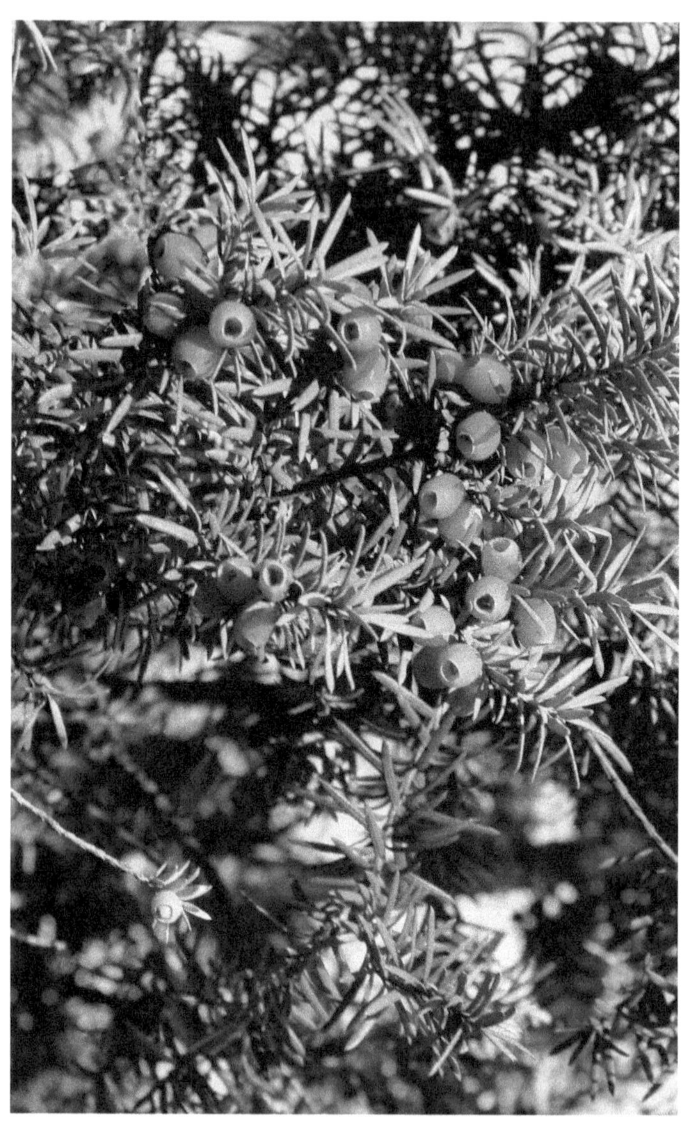

© depositphotos - Manka

yew with poisonous red fruits

Likewise, these three woodland evergreens keep their leaves in winter and doggedly cling to life. The pine may tally in the alphabet of runes with kenaz, a rune of self-realization and -protection but also of focused energies and determination. Along some stormy coasts, there are gnarled pines clinging to life, whatever the wind and weather. The power of pines can help us not to be blown away by the force of events but to remain steadfast and true to ourselves.

The spruce can live to be hundreds of years old and to grow to a height of 60 m, through its roots seldom sink deeply into the earth and its wood is relatively soft. As its roots spread out over the surface of the ground, the spruce establishes close contact with the earth while soaring into the sky, so it was said to be at home in both worlds, being on the one hand down to earth and on the other hand able to rise into the realms of higher insight.

In keeping its leaves over winter, the spruce advises us not to give up easily, but its relatively soft wood reminds us not to be obstinate. All in all, it advises us to be even-handed in our dealings with ourselves and others. As expressed by the rune wunjo, the spruce's joy in life lies under the surface. Its resin has a purifying effect and its energy help us to overcome obstacles and to heal inner wounds and traumas.

In folklore, it is said of the fir that it wears the same dress in all seasons, so the fir is not vain but content to make do with little. This speaks for its inner stability, as also shown by its long taproots. What is typical of the fir is its self-respect, letting it remain unmoved by the storms of life. Hence, the fir is said to have a protective power, showing us how to be true to ourselves, to develop inner strength and to face up to the challenges of life.

In Celtic mythology, the fir is like the spruce in being a tree of light, since they outlast the darkness of winter and the freezing cold without being bowed. Ritually, the spruce and fir were used as symbols of resurrection, the return of the sun and the reawakening of nature.

Both the spruce and the fir repel evil spirits and negative energies.

Ivy has generally a poor reputation, as it tends to over-run a garden, but in woodland it is protective. It needs little light and adapts flexibly to its surroundings. A thick green canopy of ivy offers many creatures shelter and lessens the evaporation of moisture, which can then be taken up by the roots of neighboring trees.

Ivy also shelters organisms in the earth, who loosen the soil and devour litter, freeing nutrients for the world of plants.

Ivy is so modest as to accept the support of even dead matter and thereby to flourish again without even drawing nutrients out of the soil. This is what enables it to spread continually in a garden, to drape trees or to harm walls and roofs.

But in woodland, it contributes to the whole. Its tendrils explore its surroundings and mostly find something to hold onto, however unprepossessing, till it is offered a chance to clamber up to the light or to form a flat thicket.

There is a give and take between ivy and the rest of the world of plants, who let it spread without hindrance and serve as a basis for its tendrils, while being supported in turn by the ivy. The ivy thereby leads a dual existence like the ambivalent goddess with her light and dark sides: ivy has a protective but also a destructive power. To survive, it relies on its powers of exploration and further development and is able to act as a friend or as a foe.

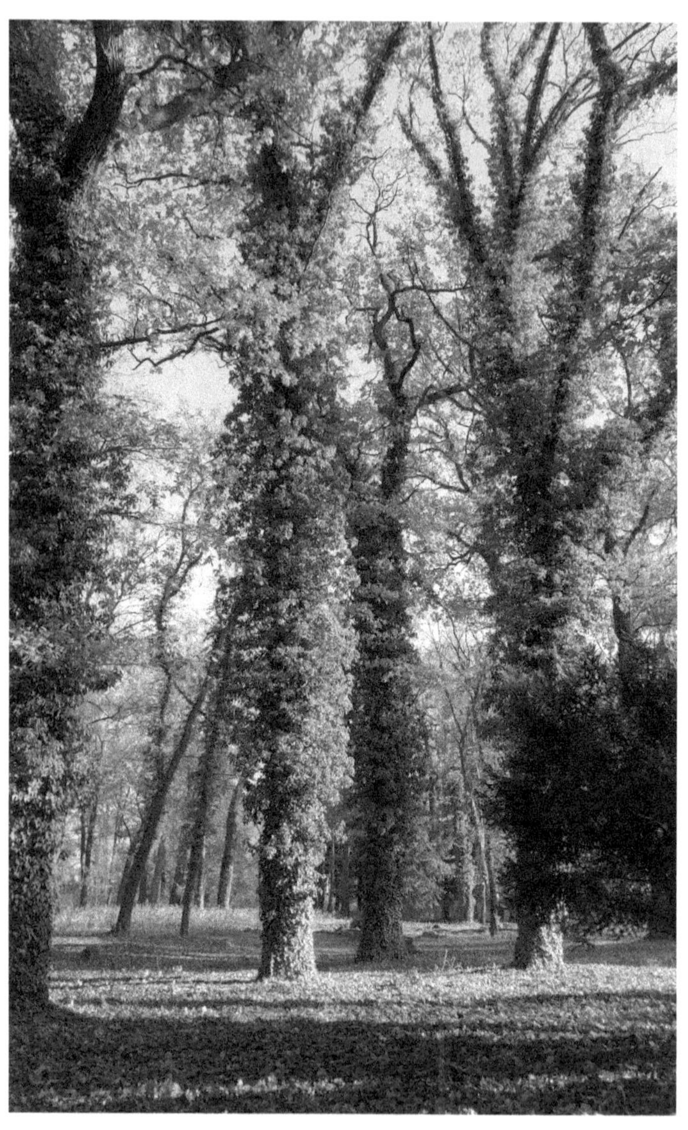

trees covered with ivy in autumn

Evergreen mistletoe is a parasite. Its seeds settle in the bark of trees then grow with the help of nutrients in the tree's sap. The various German names for mistletoe or its effect on its host's tissue reveal the magic attributed to it, the equivalents in English being druid's foot, witch's broom and elf's tendrils. Druids harvested the young shoots and slightly sickle-shaped leaves from mistletoe on oaks, taking care that the shoots harvested never touched the ground. At the yule festival at the winter solstice, mistletoe was used to decorate rooms and cult sites as a symbol of the return of the sun and light, a fresh start and the resurrection of life. Even nowadays, couples kiss each other under the mistletoe, to renew their vow of love in the hope of further happiness.

The red berries of mistletoe were said to repel witches if worn round the neck, and mistletoe itself was said to settle on trees to protect them from nightmares. More generally, it was thought to repel negative energies and curses.

Woodland spirits

The woodland is full of life, not only in the plants and trees but also in the soil and air, where the elemental spirits are at home. The elementals of air are the sylphs, those of water are the undines, those of fire are the salamanders, and those of earth are the gnomes, who are also protectors of the neighboring dimensions, together with a number of other beings. The spirits at home in the woods are called woodland spirits. Apart from the tree-spirits, there are elves, fairies, nymphs, fauns and satyrs. Some nymphs of the woodland are called dryads or meliads according to which trees they prefer, whereas hamadryads are less partial. They are all part of the invisible life of the woodland, which they also protect.

Tree-spirits are inseparable from their trees, whereas many other spirits are free to roam or to linger by certain places.

Tree-spirits may be taken to be the astral bodies of trees, just as humans have not only physical bodies but also astral ones. A tree-spirit is a being we can get in touch with by interacting with a tree. Hence a tree has an individual personality. Any tree is a certain kind of tree and has the qualities associated with its kind but is also an individual in its own right.

Dryads are associated with oaks, and meliads with ash-trees. Hamadryads are associated with individual trees, whereas dryads and meliads are not bound to linger by any one tree. Gnomes are more or less root-spirits, helping trees to draw their powers from the soil.

The use of the word fauna for animals in general reveals the nature of fauns. They are woodland spirits, often shown in half-animal form and said to cherish and protect woodland. They protect the animals there but they also protect plants, without which there could be no animals. Satyrs are similar, though apparently being more inclined to wander.

Likewise fairies and elves seem to be much the same and to differ mainly according to the culture and attitude of the beholder. Elves are beings of light, who are also lighthearted and tend to linger in tallying parts of woodland. Fairies are mistier and more translucent beings and work for the well-being and protection of woodland while being even less obtrusive.

If we open our senses, we may become aware of some of them. We may feel more lighthearted ourselves, if we happen to be in the company of elves or, if next to a tree, we may feel much the same as its spirit. Out of the corners of our eyes, we may even see a shimmer of light or a hint of mist, as the woodland spirits pass. People attuned to more ethereal planes claim to have seen more, but even the rest of us may enrich our experience of woodland by opening out minds and senses to their presence.

The winter solstice marks the longest night and shortest day of the year. From the 21st or 22nd of December, the sun begins to rise a little earlier and to set a little later each day. In heathen times, the winter solstice was also called yule. The following period is often the coldest of the year, but the sun rises higher and higher. Nature receives more warmth and light and is able to get ready for spring and a fresh start.

Darkness begins yielding to light, and coldness to warmth. This transition was celebrated by the Celts and other peoples. They used the winter solstice or the yuletide festival to appease the gods and to ask them for growth and fertility in the new year. Fires were lit and sacrifices offered.

The winter solstice also marks the start of the twelve days of Christmas. The veil between this world and the next was thought to be thinner then, so it was easier to get in touch with deceased forebears, while the spirit of winter was being chased away. Even today, there are customs dating back to these times.

Basically the winter solstice is the day when the sun is reborn. In some cultures this is the birthday of the sun-god. The fact that Christmas is now celebrated not on the 21st or 22nd but on the 25th of December is due to a change of calendar. In earlier times, calendars were aligned with the seasons differently, as shown by the twelve days of Christmas. These were days left over at the end of a year in calendars based on the moon's cycles so were like a crack in a wall, revealing a world outside.

Nature may be viewed as the source of all being and as the essence of all life. Without trees and plants, there would be no basis for our existence. People used to be well aware of this and to revere woodland as holy. Druids knew how to use the magic of trees and plants and were able to get in touch with the spirits of woodland. Shamans, too, are able to see more than meets the eye and to explore more ethereal planes.

Rituals help us to become closer to woodland and greenery and to thank them for granting us life. To take part in the rituals, we need not be druids or shamans, to call ourselves witches or to learn magic. We need only open our minds and senses and be willing to take woodland to heart.

It is already a kind of ritual to hug a tree and to thank it by watering it. We may also make keepsakes out of pieces of wood in the glades, like gnomes out of fir-cones and leaves. We may also decorate our homes with leaves, twigs and other items found on our wanderings.

If we can find a place in woodland which somehow appeals to us, we can sit down and tune into its energy or vibrant vitality by daydreaming. We need only become more keenly aware of our leafy surroundings and let them work upon us.

To practice a proper ritual, we may surround ourselves with a ring of stones or branches, to protect us symbolically from any unpleasant influences. We can now free our thoughts from all negative energies and ask the woodland for fresh and positive promptings.

We may then feel how it reacts, how the power of the earth flows through us, lifting the burdens from our shoulders and dissolving them in the air, just as superfluous water evaporates from the leaves of a tree.

We may finally thank the woodland with a small gift intuitively chosen.

If we would like to get in touch with nature spirits in the woodland, we can likewise resort to a small ritual. We can look for a small stone which appeals to us and gather some rainwater and a little sand and get hold of some incense. In woodland it is best to use incense cones, to avoid any risk of wildfire. For the same reason, it is better to use a so-called grave-light or tea-light instead of a normal candle and to place it in a fireproof glass. We can take with us another glass as well and two small dishes.

We can then choose a pleasantly restful place, fill the glass with rainwater and the dish with sand. The other dish can be filled with some loam from the earth nearby.

The candle should be placed in the glass just to the south of us and lit. The dish with sand should hold a lit incense cone and be placed to the east. The glass with rainwater should be placed to the west, and the dish with loam be placed to the north.

The items are thereby placed in directions tallying with the elements and elementals.

We should then shut our eyes and with our other senses heed everything around us as intensely as possible through scents, sounds, air and earth.

The stone is then to be taken and held over the candle-flame with the words: 'I dedicate to your the element fire.'

Then hold the stone in the smoke of the incense cone and dedicate it to the element air, then dip it in the water and dedicate it to the element water. Finally, lay it in the dish of loam and dedicate it to the element earth.

The stone should then be taken in both hands and infused with the wish to be put in touch with the woodland spirits or their energies.

We should then open our senses once more and let everything around us work intensely upon us. Our sensing is our way to get in touch with the beings, to whom we have directed our wish. We should be in no hurry but take as much time as seems to be suitable.

Finally with our fingers we should dig a small hole and put the stone into it. This is our gift for the woodland spirits. We should empty the dish of loam over the stone and offer our thanks to the beings of the earth. We should do the same with the water as well as with the remains of the cone of incense extinguished in the sand and offer our thanks to the elementals of air and earth. We should then put the candle out too and offer our thanks to the elemental of fire. Finally we should thank the woodland spirits and bid them farewell.

If we repeat the ritual now and then, the contact can become increasingly intense and clear. We can also lend free rein to our imagination, since the effectiveness of a ritual always depends on how comfortable we feel with it and how well it tallies with out natures. Maybe you can devise a little ritual of your own for use at the next winter solstice.

Old cult sites such as Stonehenge are certainly places where we can feel a special power, energy or ambiance. The same is true of many mystical places. So-called sites of power can also be found in woodland and are places where special energies flow or converge. They are places where woodland spirits feel at ease and we too may appreciate the special magic.

Sometimes the site is marked by a group of trees, a small clearing, a natural ring of stones, a spring or the bank of a brook. It is sometimes marked by the stump of a tree, a boulder or rocky ledge and sometimes by a ring of mushrooms. Often, it is enough for us to find a sheltered spot where we especially enjoy the tranquility. Such a place is very suitable for a ritual or meditation.

A site of power can be recognized through its effect on us or on the local flora. Fungi or trees may form a ring or the growth of the trees may be odd, as when a couple of trees grow into each other, or the shapes of roots are remarkable, creating passages or hollows. Sites of power differ from each other but all of them look rather strange or even remarkable. To find one, we need only wander through woodland with open eyes and ears and rely on our impressions.

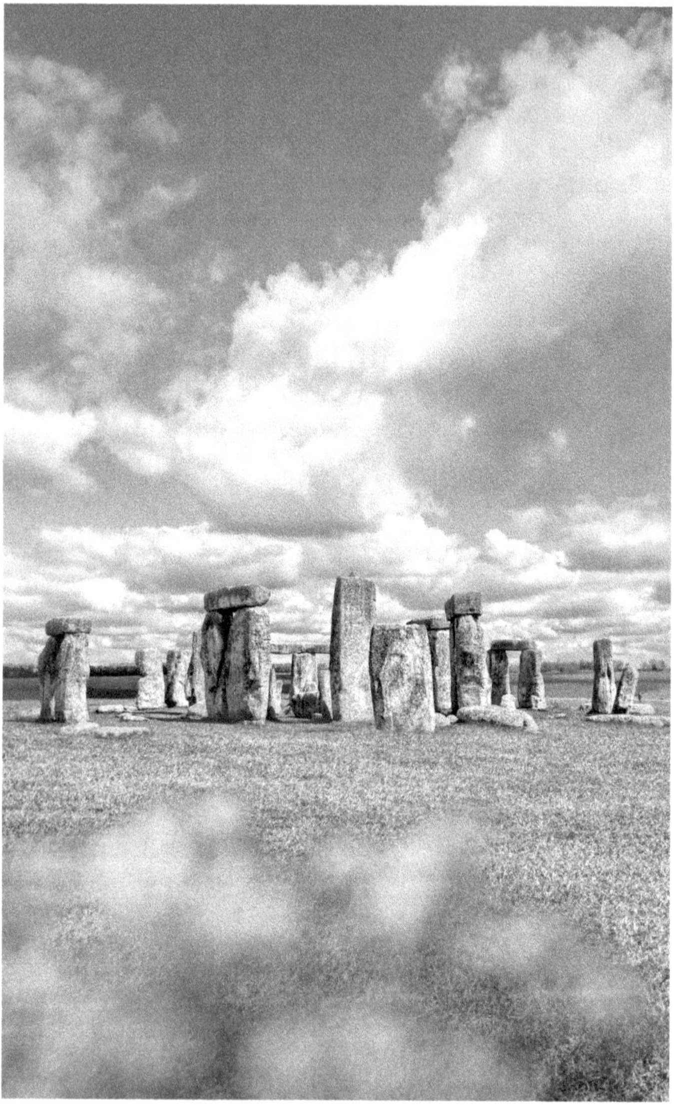

Stonehenge - southern England

122

Wandering through woodland with a partner or even with several friends may improve communication, and strolling attentively with a partner may deepen a friendship or love, but in general a stroll through woodland should be undertaken alone.

This is because strolling alone is the best way for us to revert to our roots. Only then is it possible to make the most of the chance to relax and to take in and digest all the impressions. We can focus on nature's overwhelming beauty and do it justice by heeding it fully. There is no distraction or dissipation, so we can find our ways back to our roots and become part of the woodland.

To be accepted or even welcomed by woodland is a deeply healing experience. In strolling alone through woodland, we are free to take our time and to dally wherever we feel fit. The moments of rest, the listening to soft sounds, the withdrawal from everyday life and the immersion in greenery open up new perspectives. We put one foot in front of the other, savor the here and now and the sensuousness of nature.

No-one is there to distract us with small talk or by telling us what to do. We have no need to be careful not to tread on anyone's toes. Free from any distractions, we are not disoriented but able to note the rhythm of our steps in moving along and to give free reign to our thoughts and feelings.

It is one thing to be alone and another thing to be lonely. Being alone in woodland means only keeping civilization at more than an arm's length for awhile, to do things in our own time and to appreciate the welcoming presence of nature. Tranquility and the absence of conversation are not experienced as isolation or helplessness but as a chance to relish peaceful and purifying interludes. Our minds, otherwise drawn this way and that, become calm and clear, and our thoughts fall freely into place. Old obsessions turn out to have no more worth and are easily tossed away, and our thoughts crystallize out into new patterns. Decisions are made effortlessly with the help of our intuition and the powers of nature.

Being alone is the most intense and relaxing way to be one with nature. Only alone can we appreciate it fully and draw from it new energy and power.

Be alone but never lonely!

The vitality of woodland

Woods are the earth's lungs and without them we would not be alive today. Trees and plants supply us with nutrition and ensure that the climate stays healthy and stable. But a wood is more than a gathering of trees. Apart from all the visible plants and animals, it is the home of many elementals. These are a part of woodland and care for it and protect it.

Even science has to admit that woodland is a wonder of nature, whose trees are highly evolved and social. They have sophisticated protective and defensive mechanisms, take care of and support each other and share information. They even limit the harm caused by wind by nodding their crowns separately, thereby slowing it down and letting many of them survive unscathed.

What science does not accept is that woods have souls. It realizes that plants and trees have various qualities and healing powers of use in the domain of medicine, but only a person with an open mind and heart may encounter such beings as elves, fairies, gnomes and other nature spirits.

Those of us who feel the enchantment of woodland and who yield to it and take it up into ourselves become familiar with a strange but fascinating world. There are conversations with trees, sites of special power, the energies of nature and the essence of life.

Woodland pulses with vitality and is the home of ethereal beings, which a person otherwise caught up in everyday life knows only from fairy-tales and fables. Trees are able to strengthen and comfort us, to advise us and heal us. They have souls and individual qualities, which they are only too happy to reveal to us if we let them.

But even if the hidden life of woodland remains closed to you, learn to appreciate trees and plants, because without them you would not be alive now.

**With very best wishes, your apothecary,
Dr. Angela Fetzner**

Dr. Angela Fetzner was born and grew up in Bad Kissingen in Germany. Since 1996 she has been working as a pharmacist in public and hospital pharmacies, mainly in Germany and Switzerland, and has also held seminars throughout Europe.

She qualified as a pharmacist at the Julius Maximilian University in Würzburg, went on to work for two years in a public pharmacy in the north of Germany and finally undertook postgraduate studies in the history of pharmacy at Philipps University in Marburg, gaining a doctorate (Dr. rer. Nat.).

As a trained pharmacist with useful specialized knowledge, she delights in making complex medical issues widely intelligible and since 2012 has published more than 50 guidebooks and textbooks, many of which are about healthcare and have inspired hundreds of thousands of readers.

In her spare time, she loves to withdraw into nature and to go for long walks with her donkeys, Achiel and Harrie, whom she saved from the slaughterhouse.

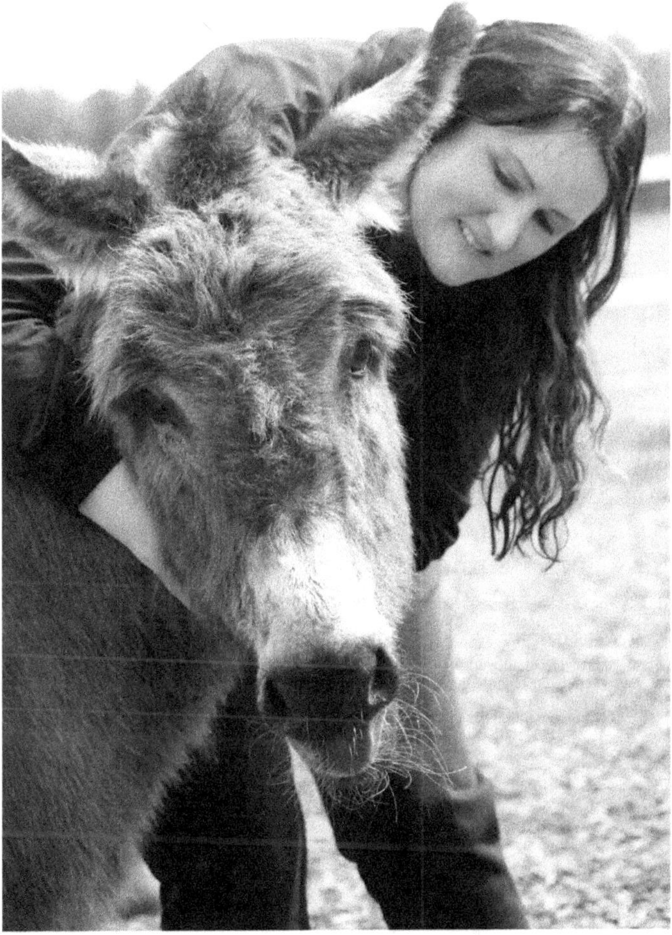

© Michael Raab

Dr. Angela Fetzner with her donkey „Harrie“

is due at this point to all my esteemed readers. If my guide has been satisfying and useful to you, I would appreciate a short review. Praise, blame or suggestions can be left on my Facebook page:

https://www.facebook.com/AngelaFetzner

or on my homepage as an author:
https://www.angela-fetzner.de

Books from Dr. Angela Fetzner
are likewise all to be found on my homepage as an author:
https://www.angela-fetzner.de
I would also like to offer my readers a special service.
My online readings are regularly announced on my homepage, where book reviews and blog articles appear too. On it, you may sign up for my newsletter for regular information about new books, promotions and raffles as well as health tips.
My e-books are in all the leading online stores, and my printed books are in the mail order and standard book trade. I myself am on the social networks: Facebook, Twitter, Instagram and

Youtube: https://angela-fetzner.de//

Dr. Angela Fetzner

The Lymph
The Body's Purification Plant

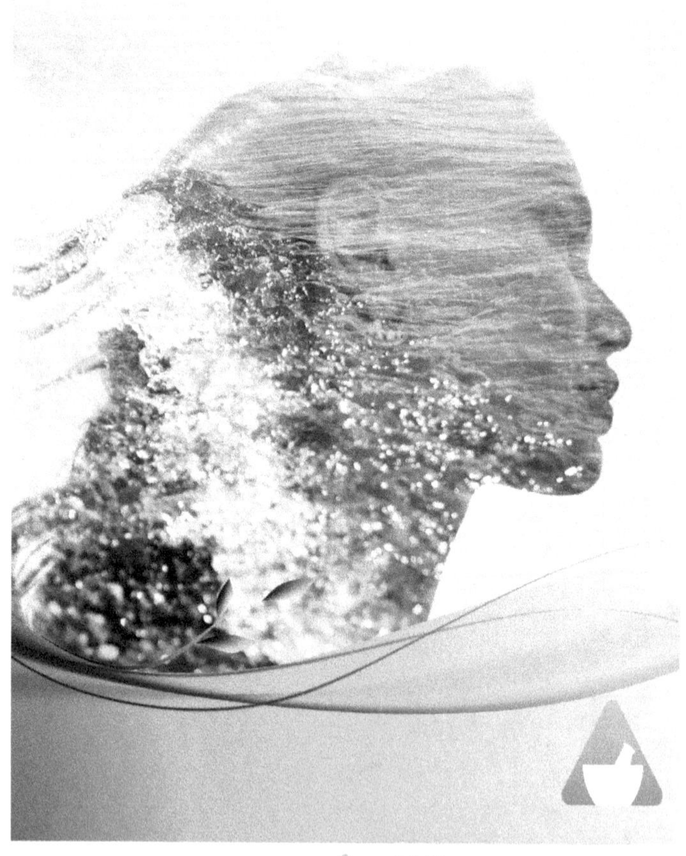

Lymphatic cleansing

This has become the stepchild of all detoxification therapy. Cleansing of the liver or colon is high on the agenda, but detoxification of the lymphatic system is often neglected. Regular detoxification of the lymphatic system is nonetheless crucial for physical and mental health.

The lymphatic system

This is the body's purification plant, ridding it of whatever is harmful or useless like pathogens, metabolic waste, toxins and cell debris. It is crucial for immunity and the body's detoxification.

Sustaining the flow

The lymphatic system must be regularly cleansed and detoxified to keep on flowing naturally. If continually overloaded with waste, it stagnates. The system can no longer get rid of all problematic materials, so these gradually poison the whole body and often cause chronic ailments.

Lymphatic cleansing

This book outlines all natural therapies and treatments which have proven to be effective in basic lymphatic detoxification and cleansing. These everyday ways to look after yourself are motivating and efficient. They include approaches like medicinal plant therapy, homeopathy, Schuessler salts, specific cleansing of the lymph, water applications, stress reduction, changes of diet, moderate exercise and so on. With the help of these choice means of detoxification, you will soon feel livelier, stronger and merrier.

As a doctor of pharmacology, the author has been advising and informing clients for more than two decades, being committed to their health and well being.

Your pharmacist, Angela Fetzner

Dr. Angela Fetzner

Power Animals & Shamanism

Finding the Lost Soul

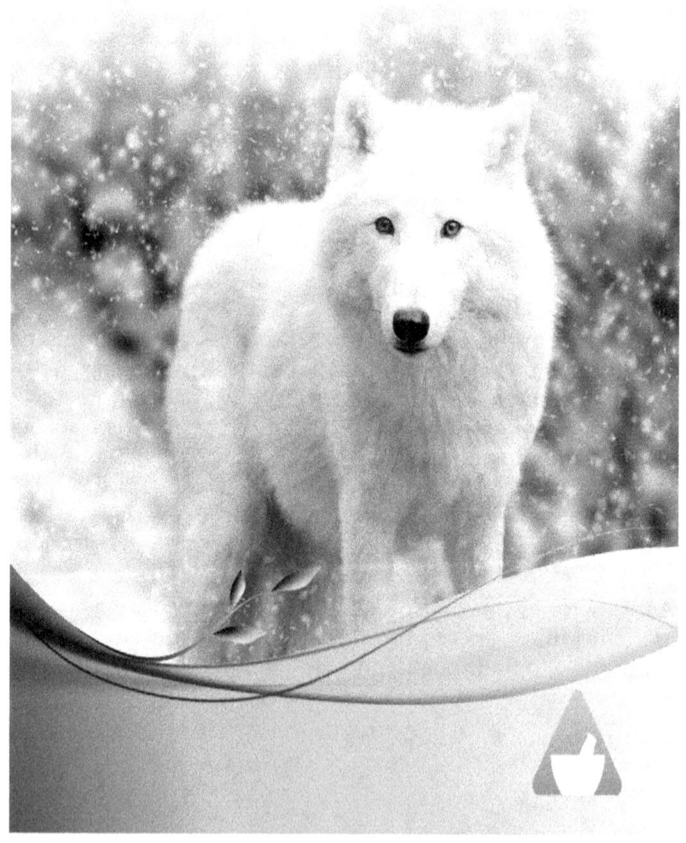

Regaining a lost soul

In this book, the millennia-old healing techniques of shamanism are presented clearly and appealingly. The book is meant to give readers an overview of the complex and manifold facets of shamanism and to encourage them to reach out to their respective power animal.

Power animals – spiritual companions and leaders

Power animals are spiritual companions and soulmates, and each has a personal relationship with its human counterpart, who is thereby empowered, energized, deepened and motivated. The person is enabled to find his or her true purpose, to develop more fully and to avoid pitfalls, is protected, kept healthy and even healed, and can turn to the animal for help at any time. The more he or she does so, the more intense their partnership becomes. Some partnerships last a lifetime.

How do you find your power animal?

This book explains how to find, honor and bond with your power animal and thereby be strengthened and healed. It explains how the animal may be lost and how the loss may be averted.

The main power animals

The most important power animals and their meaning and message for humans are discussed in detail, revealing what positive qualities may be transferred from one to you.

The worldview of shamanism

This book offers all key information about shamanism and how to use it. The division of the shamanic cosmos into the upper, middle and lower worlds is explained, as are details of shamanic journeys. The role of the master of animals in particular is examined, as is the difference between spirit helpers and totem animals. The basic features of neo-shamanism are shown too.

Detoxification – the removal of pollutants from the body – can look back on a long tradition.

Since time immemorial, people have felt a wish to cleanse their bodies and souls at regular intervals and to rid them of needless and harmful ballast. This may be due to the instinctive feeling that purification is a great relief for body and soul and is also needed to maintain or regain health. At the same time, a thorough detoxification and cleansing of the body is a prerequisite for all deeper processes of healing.

Among other things, detoxification measures are used to activate the body's powers of self-healing. Only by thoroughly removing pollutants can we remove the precondition for many ailments, letting body and soul recover.

This book describes all natural therapies which have proven to be effective in basic detoxification. These measures are down to earth, motivating and efficient and include medicinal plant therapy, homeopathy, Schuessler salts, specific cleansing of the organs of detoxification, water applications, wraps, reduction of stress, changes of diet and so on.

With the help of the detoxification cures here chosen and presented, you will soon regain your vitality, strength and zeal.

With kind regards from your pharmacist, Dr. Angela Fetzner